MW01609753

Table of Contents

4

8

Introduction

Many conditions cause inflammation and this ailment could harm your overall health and state of being. If you are one of the many people who suffer from such a condition and you need to find an improvement, you might need to consider changing your eating habits.

Experts in the field have developed an interesting diet that decreases inflammation and, in turn, makes significant improvements in your health.

This great diet is extremely healthy and easy to follow as long as you follow some basic principles. You will see its benefits quite quickly and you will feel and look amazing!

If you decide to follow an anti-inflammatory diet, you need to give up eating certain foods and start consuming others that contain anti-inflammatory elements.

So, here's what you *can* eat on an anti-inflammatory diet.

To begin, you have to start eating more veggies and fruits. While you should consume all kind of veggies, you should especially eat a lot of leafy greens such as kale or spinach and also cabbage and broccoli. Fruits like berries, cherries, apples and pears will also be very beneficial to easing your inflammation.

Eating more whole grains like rice, oatmeal and others that contain a lot of healthy fibers will also help you to feel better. And don't forget about eating more beans, nuts, healthy oils, fish, poultry and some pork too!

Last but not least, if you are on an anti-inflammatory diet, you need to consume a lot of herbs and spices that will help decrease inflammation. We recommend you to start using a lot of garlic, curry, turmeric, chili powder and saffron in preparing your meals as all of these have been proven to help with inflammation.

Now, that you know what to eat on an anti-inflammatory diet you should also know what not to eat.

Well, this part is pretty simple. Essentially, you are not allowed to consume processed foods, greasy foods or very sweet ones. You can no longer eat refined starches, processed red meat or dairy products.

As you can see, it's rather simple to follow an anti-inflammatory diet. Just focus on your goals, stick to the foods that are beneficial and get your hands on a copy of our anti-inflammatory cookbook!

This way you will be able to start a new and healthy life in no time!

So, what are you waiting for? Start following an anti-inflammatory diet today and enjoy life!

Breakfast Recipes

Blueberry Smoothie

Preparation time: 10 minutes
Cooking time: 0 minutes
Servings: 1

Ingredients:

- 1 banana, peeled
- 2 handfuls baby spinach
- 1 tablespoon almond butter
- ½ cup blueberries
- ¼ teaspoon ground cinnamon
- 1 teaspoon maca powder
- ½ cup water
- ½ cup almond milk, unsweetened

Directions:
In your blender, mix the spinach with the banana, blueberries, almond butter, cinnamon, maca powder, water and milk. Pulse well, pour into a glass and serve.
Enjoy!

Nutrition: calories 341, fat 12, fiber 11, carbs 54, protein 10

Delicious Amaranth Porridge

Preparation time: 10 minutes
Cooking time: 30 minutes
Servings: 2

Ingredients:

- ½ cup water
- 1 cup almond milk, unsweetened
- ½ cup amaranth
- 1 pear, peeled and cubed
- ½ teaspoon ground cinnamon
- ¼ teaspoon fresh ginger, grated
- A pinch of ground nutmeg
- 1 teaspoon maple syrup
- 2 tablespoons chopped pecans

Directions:
Put the water and the almond milk in a pot, bring to a simmer over medium heat, add the amaranth, mix and cook for 20 minutes. Add the pear, cinnamon, ginger, nutmeg and maple syrup and mix. Simmer for 10 minutes more, divide into bowls and serve with pecans sprinkled on top.
Enjoy!

Nutrition: calories 199, fat 9, fiber 4, carbs 25, protein 3

Breakfast Salad

Preparation time: 10 minutes
Cooking time: 0 minutes
Servings: 4

Ingredients:

- 27 ounces kale salad mixed with dried fruit
- 1 ½ cups blueberries
- 15 ounces beets, cooked, peeled and cubed
- ¼ cup olive oil
- 2 tablespoons apple cider vinegar
- 1 teaspoon turmeric powder
- 1 tablespoon lemon juice
- 1 garlic clove, minced
- 1 teaspoon fresh grated ginger
- A pinch of black pepper

Directions:
In a salad bowl, mix the kale and dried fruit with beets and blueberries. In a separate bowl, mix the oil with the vinegar, turmeric, lemon juice, garlic, ginger and a pinch of black pepper, whisk well then pour over the salad, toss and serve.
Enjoy!

Nutrition: calories 188, fat 4, fiber 6, carbs 14, protein 7

Sweet Potato Breakfast Salad

Preparation time: 10 minutes
Cooking time: 0 minutes
Servings: 2

Ingredients:

- 1 scoop protein powder
- ¼ cup blueberries
- ¼ cup raspberries
- 1 banana, peeled
- 1 sweet potato, baked, peeled and cubed

Directions:
Put the potato in a bowl and mash it with a fork. Add banana and protein powder and mix everything together well. Add the berries, mix and serve cold.
Enjoy!

Nutrition: calories 181, fat 1, fiber 6, carbs 8, protein 11

Delicious Turmeric Milk

Preparation time: 10 minutes
Cooking time: 5 minutes
Servings: 2

Ingredients:

- 1½ cups coconut milk, unsweetened
- 1½ cups almond milk, unsweetened
- ¼ teaspoon ground ginger
- 1½ teaspoon ground turmeric
- 1 tablespoon coconut oil
- ¼ teaspoon ground cinnamon

Directions:
Put the coconut and almond milk in a small pot and heat over medium heat, add the ginger, oil, turmeric and cinnamon. Mix and cook for 5 minutes, divide into bowls and serve.
Enjoy!

Nutrition: calories 171, fat 3, fiber 4, carbs 6, protein 7

Almond Oats

Preparation time: 10 minutes
Cooking time: 0 minutes
Servings: 2

Ingredients:

- 1 cup old-fashioned oats
- ½ cup coconut milk
- 1 tablespoon maple syrup
- ¼ cup blueberries
- 3 tablespoons chopped almonds

Directions:
In a bowl, mix the oats with the coconut milk, maple syrup and almonds. Cover and let sit overnight. Serve the following day.
Enjoy!

Nutrition: calories 255, fat 9, fiber 6, carbs 39, protein 7

Turmeric Chocolate

Preparation time: 10 minutes
Cooking time: 5 minutes
Servings: 2

Ingredients:

- 1 cup coconut milk, unsweetened
- 2 teaspoons coconut oil, melted
- 1½ tablespoons cocoa powder
- 1 teaspoon ground turmeric
- A pinch of black pepper
- A pinch of cayenne pepper
- 2 teaspoons raw honey

Directions:
Put the milk in a pan, heat it over medium heat, add the oil, cocoa powder, turmeric, black pepper, cayenne and honey. Whisk well, cook for 5 minutes, pour into a cup and serve. Enjoy!

Nutrition: calories 281, fat 12, fiber 4, carbs 12, protein 7

Turkey Hash

Preparation time: 10 minutes
Cooking time: 15 minutes
Servings: 4

Ingredients:

- 1 pound ground turkey
- ½ teaspoon dried thyme
- 1 tablespoon coconut oil, melted
- ½ teaspoon ground cinnamon

For the hash:

- 1 yellow onion, chopped
- 1 tablespoon coconut oil, melted
- 1 zucchini, chopped
- ½ cup shredded carrots
- 2 cups butternut squash, cubed
- 1 apple, cored, peeled and cubed
- 2 cups baby spinach
- 1 teaspoon ground ginger
- 1 teaspoon ground cinnamon
- ½ teaspoon garlic powder
- ½ teaspoon turmeric powder
- ½ teaspoon dried thyme

Directions:
Heat up a pan with 1 tablespoon coconut oil over medium-high heat. Add the turkey, ½ teaspoon thyme and ½ teaspoon ground cinnamon. Mix and cook for 5 minutes then transfer to a bowl. Heat up the pan again with 1 tablespoon coconut oil over medium-high heat. Add the onion, stir and cook for 2 minutes. Add the zucchini, the carrots, squash, apple, ginger, 1 teaspoon cinnamon, ½ teaspoon thyme, turmeric and garlic powder. Stir and cook for 3-4 minutes. Return the meat to the pan, also add the baby spinach. Mix together and cook for 1-2 minutes more then divide everything between plates and serve for breakfast.
Enjoy!

Nutrition: calories 212, fat 4, fiber 6, carbs 8, protein 7

Tropical Bowls

Preparation time: 10 minutes
Cooking time: 0 minutes
Servings: 2

Ingredients:
- 1 cup orange juice
- 1 cup mango, peeled and cubed
- 1 cup pineapple, peeled and cubed
- 1 banana, peeled
- 1 teaspoon chia seeds
- A pinch of turmeric powder
- 4 strawberries, sliced

Directions:
In your blender, mix the orange juice with the mango, pineapple, banana, chia seeds and turmeric. Pulse well, divide into bowls, top each with the strawberries and serve.
Enjoy!

Nutrition: calories 171, fat 3, fiber 6, carbs 8, protein 11

Beet Smoothie

Preparation time: 10 minutes
Cooking time: 0 minutes
Servings: 2

Ingredients:
- 10 ounces almond milk, unsweetened
- 2 beets, peeled and quartered
- ½ banana, peeled and frozen
- ½ cup cherries, pitted
- 1 tablespoon almond butter

Directions:
In your blender, mix the milk with the beets, banana, cherries and butter. Pulse well, pour into glasses and serve.
Enjoy!

Nutrition: calories 165, fat 5, fiber 6, carbs 22, protein 5

Chia Bars

Preparation time: 4 hours
Cooking time: 0 minutes
Servings: 4

Ingredients:
- 1½ cups dates, pitted and chopped
- ½ cup chia seeds
- 1/3 cup cocoa powder
- ½ cup shredded coconut, unsweetened
- 1 cup chopped walnuts
- ½ cup oats
- ½ cup dark chocolate, chopped
- 1 teaspoon vanilla extract

Directions:
In your food processor, mix the dates with the chia seeds, cocoa, coconut, walnuts, oats, chocolate and vanilla. Pulse well then press into a lined baking dish. Keep in the freezer for 4 hours, cut into 12 bars and serve for breakfast.
Enjoy!

Nutrition: calories 125, fat 5, fiber 4, carbs 12, protein 5

Green Eggs Mix

Preparation time: 10 minutes
Cooking time: 30 minutes
Servings: 4

Ingredients:
- 2 garlic cloves, minced
- 1 pound spinach, torn
- 2 tablespoons olive oil
- 1 yellow onion, chopped
- 1 jalapeno, chopped
- 1 teaspoon cumin, dried
- A pinch of salt and black pepper
- 1 teaspoon coriander, ground
- 2 tablespoons harissa
- ½ cup veggie stock
- 8 eggs
- 1 tablespoon cilantro, chopped
- 1 tablespoon parsley, chopped

Directions:
Heat up a pan with the oil over medium heat, add the onion, stir and cook for 4 minutes. Add the jalapeno and the garlic, stir and cook for a few more seconds. Add the spinach, stir and cook for 4 minutes. Add salt, pepper, harissa, coriander and cumin. Cook for 1 minute, transfer to your food processor, add the stock then pulse well, return the mix to the pan and spread it well. Make 8 holes in this mix and crack an egg in each hole. Place the dish in the oven, bake at 350 degrees F for 20 minutes, divide between plates, sprinkle cilantro and parsley on top and serve.
Enjoy!

Nutrition: calories 251, fat 12, fiber 4, carbs 12, protein 14

Chia Pudding

Preparation time: 4 hours
Cooking time: 0 minutes
Servings: 3

Ingredients:

- 2 cups coconut milk, unsweetened
- 1 banana, peeled and sliced
- ½ cup chia seeds
- ½ teaspoon vanilla extract
- 2 tablespoon raw honey
- 1 tablespoon cocoa powder
- 2 tablespoon cocoa nibs

Directions:
In a bowl, mix the banana with the chia seeds, and mash using a fork. Add the milk, the vanilla extract, honey, cocoa powder and cocoa nibs, mix and keep in the fridge for 4 hours before serving.
Enjoy!

Nutrition: calories 313, fat 14, fiber 17, carbs 36, protein 10

Pineapple Smoothie

Preparation time: 10 minutes
Cooking time: 0 minutes
Servings: 1

Ingredients:

- 1 cup coconut water
- 1 orange, peeled and cut into quarters
- 1½ cups pineapple chunks
- 1 tablespoon fresh grated ginger
- 1 teaspoon chia seeds
- 1 teaspoon turmeric powder
- A pinch of black pepper

Directions:
In your blender, mix the coconut water with the orange, pineapple, ginger, chia seeds, turmeric and black pepper. Pulse well, pour into a glass and serve for breakfast.
Enjoy!

Nutrition: calories 151, fat 2, fiber 6, carbs 12, protein 4

Porridge

Preparation time: 10 minutes
Cooking time: 5 minutes
Servings: 2

Ingredients:

- ¼ cup walnuts, chopped and toasted
- 2 tablespoons hemp seeds, toasted
- 2 tablespoons chia seeds
- 1 cup almond milk, unsweetened
- ¼ cup coconut milk, unsweetened
- ¼ cup coconut, shredded and toasted
- ¼ cup almond butter
- 1 tablespoon coconut oil, melted
- ½ teaspoon turmeric powder
- 1 teaspoon bee pollen
- A pinch of black pepper

Directions:
Heat up a pot with the almond and coconut milk over medium heat, add the walnuts, hemp seeds, chia seeds, coconut, turmeric, black pepper and the bee pollen, stir, cook for 5 minutes. Take off heat, add the coconut oil and the almond butter, stir and let sit for 10 minutes then divide into 2 bowls and serve.
Enjoy!

Nutrition: calories 152, fat 11, fiber 6, carbs 15, protein 11

Cucumber and Pineapple Smoothie

Preparation time: 10 minutes
Cooking time: 0 minutes
Servings: 2

Ingredients:

- 2 cups kale, torn
- 1 cup brewed green tea
- 1 cup pineapple chunks
- 1 cup cucumber, peeled and chopped
- ½ cup mango chunks, frozen
- ½ banana, peeled
- 1 teaspoon ground ginger
- ¼ teaspoon ground turmeric
- 3 mint leaves, chopped
- 1 tablespoon chia seeds
- 4 ice cubes
- 1 scoop protein powder

Directions:
In your blender, mix the kale with the green tea, pineapple, cucumber, mango, banana, ginger, turmeric, mint, protein powder and ice. Pulse well then add the chia seeds. Stir, divide into 2 glasses and serve.
Enjoy!

Nutrition: calories 161, fat 2, fiber 6, carbs 11, protein 5

Quinoa Porridge

Preparation time: 10 minutes
Cooking time: 0 minutes
Servings: 2

Ingredients:

- 1 cup cashew milk, warm
- 1 cup blueberries
- 2 cups quinoa, cooked
- ¼ cup chopped walnuts, toasted
- 2 teaspoons raw honey
- ½ teaspoon ground cinnamon
- 1 tablespoon chia seeds

Directions:
In a bowl, mix the cashew milk with the blueberries, quinoa, walnuts, honey, cinnamon and chia seeds. Stir well, divide into 2 small bowls and serve.
Enjoy!

Nutrition: calories 151, fat 2, fiber 11, carbs 14, protein 13

Raspberry Smoothie

Preparation time: 10 minutes
Cooking time: 0 minutes
Servings: 2

Ingredients:

- 1 avocado, pitted and peeled
- ¾ cup raspberry juice
- ¾ cup orange juice
- ½ cup raspberries

Directions:
In your blender, mix the avocado with the raspberry juice, orange juice and raspberries. Pulse well, divide into 2 glasses and serve.
Enjoy!

Nutrition: calories 125, fat 11, fiber 7, carbs 9, protein 3

Gingerbread Oatmeal

Preparation time: 10 minutes
Cooking time: 15 minutes
Servings: 4

Ingredients:

- 1 cup steel cut oats
- 4 cups water
- ¼ teaspoon ground coriander
- 1½ tablespoons ground cinnamon
- ¼ teaspoon ground cloves
- ¼ teaspoon fresh grated ginger
- ¼ teaspoon ground allspice
- ¼ teaspoon ground cardamom
- A pinch of ground nutmeg

Directions:

Heat up a pan with the water over medium-high heat, add the oats and stir. Add the coriander, cinnamon, cloves, ginger, allspice, cardamom and nutmeg, stir, cook for 15 minutes, divide into bowls and serve.
Enjoy!

Nutrition: calories 188, fat 3, fiber 6, carbs 13, protein 6

Rhubarb Muffins

Preparation time: 10 minutes
Cooking time: 25 minutes
Servings: 8

Ingredients:

- ½ cup almond meal
- 2 tablespoons crystallized ginger
- ¼ cup stevia
- 1 tablespoon linseed meal
- ½ cup buckwheat flour
- ¼ cup brown rice flour
- 2 tablespoons powdered arrowroot
- 2 teaspoon gluten-free baking powder
- ½ teaspoon fresh grated ginger
- ½ teaspoon ground cinnamon
- 1 cup rhubarb, sliced
- 1 apple, cored, peeled and chopped
- 1/3 cup almond milk, unsweetened
- ¼ cup olive oil
- 1 free-range egg
- 1 teaspoon vanilla extract

Directions:

In a bowl, mix the almond meal with the crystallized ginger, stevia, linseed meal, buckwheat flour, rice flour, arrowroot powder, grated ginger, baking powder and cinnamon and stir. In another bowl, mix the rhubarb with the apple, almond milk, oil, egg and vanilla and stir well. Combine the 2 mixtures, stir well, and divide into a lined muffin tray. Place in the oven at 350 degrees F and bake for 25 minutes. Serve the muffins for breakfast.
Enjoy!

Nutrition: calories 200, fat 4, fiber 6, carbs 13, protein 8

Winter Fruit Salad

Preparation time: 10 minutes
Cooking time: 0 minutes
Servings: 6

Ingredients:

- 4 persimmons, cubed
- 4 pears, cubed
- 1 cup grapes, halved
- 1 cup apples, peeled, cored and cubed
- ¾ cup pecans, halved
- 1 tablespoon olive oil
- 1 tablespoon peanut oil
- 1 tablespoon pomegranate flavored vinegar
- 2 tablespoons agave nectar

Directions:
In a salad bowl, mix the persimmons with the pears, grapes, apples and pecans. In another bowl, mix the olive oil with the peanut oil, vinegar and agave nectar. Whisk well then pour over the salad, toss and serve for breakfast.
Enjoy!

Nutrition: calories 125, fat 3, fiber 6, carbs 14, protein 8

Buckwheat Granola

Preparation time: 10 minutes
Cooking time: 45 minutes
Servings: 6

Ingredients:

- 2 cups oats
- 1 cup buckwheat
- 1 cup sunflower seeds
- 1 cup pumpkin seeds
- 1½ cups dates, pitted and chopped
- 1 cup apple puree
- 6 tablespoons coconut oil
- 5 tablespoons cocoa powder
- 1 teaspoon fresh grated ginger

Directions:
In a large bowl, mix the oats with the buckwheat, sunflower seeds, pumpkin seeds, dates, apple puree, oil, cocoa powder and ginger then stir really well. Spread on a lined baking sheet, press well and place in the oven at 360 degrees F for 45 minutes. Leave the granola to cool down, slice and serve for breakfast.
Enjoy!

Nutrition: calories 161, fat 3, fiber 5, carbs 11, protein 7

Mushroom Frittata

Preparation time: 10 minutes
Cooking time: 30 minutes
Servings: 4

Ingredients:

- ¼ cup coconut milk, unsweetened
- 6 eggs
- 1 yellow onion, chopped
- 4 ounces white mushrooms, sliced
- 2 tablespoons olive oil
- 2 cups baby spinach
- A pinch of salt and black pepper

Directions:
Heat up a pan with the oil over medium-high heat, add the onion, stir and cook for 2-3 minutes. Add the mushrooms, salt and pepper, stir and cook for 2 minutes more. In a bowl, mix the eggs with salt and pepper, stir well and pour over the mushrooms. Add the spinach, mix a bit, place in the oven and bake at 360 degrees F for 25 minutes. Slice the frittata and serve it for breakfast. Enjoy!

Nutrition: calories 200, fat 3, fiber 6, carbs 14, protein 6

Breakfast Crepes

Preparation time: 10 minutes
Cooking time: 10 minutes
Servings: 4

Ingredients:

- 2 eggs
- 1 teaspoon vanilla extract
- ½ cup almond milk, unsweetened
- ½ cup water
- 2 tablespoons agave nectar
- 1 cup coconut flour
- 3 tablespoons coconut oil, melted

Directions:
In a bowl, whisk the eggs with the vanilla extract, almond milk, water and agave nectar. Add the flour and 2 tablespoons oil gradually and stir until you obtain a smooth batter. Heat up a pan with the rest of the oil over medium heat, add some of the batter, spread into the pan and cook the crepe until it's golden on both sides then transfer to a plate. Repeat with the rest of the batter and serve the crepes for breakfast.
Enjoy!

Nutrition: calories 121, fat 3, fiber 6, carbs 14, protein 6

Millet Muffins

Preparation time: 10 minutes
Cooking time: 15 minutes
Servings: 12

Ingredients:

- ¼ cup coconut oil, melted
- 1 egg
- ½ teaspoon vanilla extract
- 1 teaspoon baking powder
- 1½ cups organic millet, cooked
- ½ cup raw honey
- Cooking spray

Directions:

In a blender, blend the melted coconut oil with the egg, vanilla extract, baking powder, millet and honey. Grease a muffin tray with cooking spray and divide the millet mix into each cup. Place the muffins in the oven and bake at 350 degrees F for 30 minutes. Let the muffins cool and then serve! Enjoy!

Nutrition: calories 167, fat 4, fiber 7, carbs 15, protein 6

Kale Smoothie

Preparation time: 10 minutes
Cooking time: 0 minutes
Servings: 5

Ingredients:

- 10 kale leaves
- 5 bananas, peeled and cut into chunks
- 2 pears, chopped
- 5 tablespoons almond butter
- 5 cups almond milk

Directions:

In your blender, mix the kale with the bananas, pears, almond butter and almond milk, pulse well, divide into glasses and serve for breakfast.
Enjoy!

Nutrition: calories 267, fat 11, fiber 7, carbs 15, protein 7

Apple Muesli

Preparation time: 10 minutes
Cooking time: 0 minutes
Servings: 4

Ingredients:

- 2 apples, peeled, cored and grated
- 1 cup rolled oats
- 3 tablespoons flax seeds
- 1¼ cups coconut cream
- 1¼ cups coconut water
- ½ cup goji berries
- 2 tablespoons chopped mint
- 3 tablespoons raw honey

Directions:
In a bowl, mix the apples with the oats, flax seeds, coconut cream, coconut water, goji berries, mint and honey. Stir well, divide into smaller bowls and serve for breakfast.
Enjoy!

Nutrition: calories 171, fat 2, fiber 6, carbs 14, protein 5

Veggie and Onion Mix

Preparation time: 10 minutes
Cooking time: 10 minutes
Servings: 2

Ingredients:

- ½ cup chopped yellow onions
- ½ cup chopped red bell pepper
- A pinch of garlic powder
- A pinch of salt and black pepper
- 1 tablespoon olive oil
- 2 eggs

Directions:
Heat up a pan with the oil over medium-high heat, add the onions, stir and cook for 1-2 minutes. Add the bell pepper, garlic powder, salt and pepper then stir and cook for 3 minutes more. Add the eggs, stir and cook until the eggs are done, about 1-2 minutes. Divide everything between plates and serve.
Enjoy!

Nutrition: calories 221, fat 6, fiber 6, carbs 14, protein 11

Sweet Potato Cakes

Preparation time: 10 minutes
Cooking time: 10 minutes
Servings: 6

Ingredients:

- 1 cup coconut flour
- 2 tablespoons brown rice flour
- ½ tablespoon ground flax seed
- 1 teaspoon baking soda
- A pinch of salt and black pepper
- 3 eggs
- 1 small yellow onion, chopped
- 2 garlic cloves, minced
- 1 small sweet potato, peeled and grated
- 2½ cups chopped kale
- 3 tablespoons olive oil

Directions:
In a bowl, add the coconut flour with the rice flour, flax seed, baking soda, salt, pepper, eggs, onion, garlic, sweet potato and kale stir well. Shape medium cakes out of this mix, you should get about 6 cakes. Heat up a pan with the olive oil over medium-high heat then add the cakes and cook them for about 4-5 minutes on each side. Divide them between plates and serve them for breakfast.
Enjoy!

Nutrition: calories 211, fat 4, fiber 7, carbs 14, protein 7

Healthy Salad

Preparation time: 10 minutes
Cooking time: 0 minutes
Servings: 2

Ingredients:

- 1 cucumber, sliced
- 2 handfuls cherry tomatoes, halved
- 1 avocado, peeled, pitted and cubed
- 1 red bell pepper, cubed
- A handful basil, torn
- A handful parsley, chopped
- 1 tablespoon olive oil
- ¼ cup pine nuts, toasted
- A pinch of salt and black pepper

Directions:
In a salad bowl, mix the cucumber with the cherry tomatoes, avocado, bell pepper, basil, parsley, salt, pepper, oil and pine nuts. Toss the mix together then divide between plates and serve for breakfast.
Enjoy!

Nutrition: calories 181, fat 4, fiber 4, carbs 11, protein 5

Bean Sprout Breakfast Salad

Preparation time: 10 minutes
Cooking time: 2 minutes
Servings: 2

Ingredients:

- 1½ cups mixed bean sprouts, soaked for 12 hours and drained
- 1/3 cup tomato, cubed
- 1/3 cup carrot, grated
- 1 cucumber, sliced
- ½ cup yellow onion, chopped
- 10 mint leaves, chopped
- 1 tablespoon olive oil
- 1 tablespoon chaat masala
- 1 tablespoon lemon juice
- A pinch of salt and black pepper

Directions:
Heat up a pan with the oil over medium-high heat, add the bean sprouts, toss and cook for 1 minute. Add the tomato, carrot, cucumber, onion, mint, chaat masala, lemon juice, salt and pepper then toss and cook for 1-2 minutes more. Divide into bowls and serve for breakfast. Enjoy!

Nutrition: calories 177, fat 2, fiber 6, carbs 15. protein 6

Fruit and Veggie Breakfast Mix

Preparation time: 10 minutes
Cooking time: 0 minutes
Servings: 3

Ingredients:

- 1 cup baby spinach, torn
- 6 lettuce leaves, torn
- 1 peach, chopped
- 1 mango, cubed
- 1 cucumber, sliced
- 10 strawberries, halved
- 1 tablespoon hemp seeds
- 1 tablespoon tahini paste
- 1 tablespoon lime juice
- 1 tablespoon coconut water
- 1 teaspoon dates, chopped
- ½ teaspoon spirulina powder

Directions:
In a bowl, mix the tahini paste with the lime juice, water, dates and spirulina, stir well. In a separate salad bowl, mix the spinach with the lettuce, peach, mango, cucumber, strawberries and hemp seeds. Toss the salad together then add the salad dressing and toss again. Serve for breakfast.
Enjoy!

Nutrition: calories 143, fat 2, fiber 4, carbs 30, protein 4

Rosemary Oats

Preparation time: 10 minutes
Cooking time: 15 minutes
Servings: 2

Ingredients:

- ½ cup oats
- ½ cup almond milk, unsweetened
- ½ cup water
- ½ teaspoon coconut oil, melted
- ½ cup chopped onion
- ½ cup sliced white mushrooms
- ½ cup chopped collard greens
- ½ cup chopped tomato
- ½ tablespoon chopped rosemary
- A pinch of salt and black pepper

Directions:
Heat up a pan with the coconut oil over medium-high heat. Add the onion, stir and cook for 1-2 minutes. Add the mushrooms, the collard greens, tomato, rosemary, salt and pepper, stir and cook for 5 minutes more then take off the heat. Heat up a small pot with the almond milk and the water over medium heat. Add the oats, stir and cook for 4-5 minutes. Add the collard greens mix to the pan with the oats, stir and cook for 5 minutes more. Divide into bowls and serve for breakfast.
Enjoy!

Nutrition: calories 211, fat 3, fiber 6, carbs 15, protein 7

Swiss Chard Bowls

Preparation time: 10 minutes
Cooking time: 5 minutes
Servings: 4

Ingredients:

- 1 bunch Swiss chard, chopped
- 1 garlic clove, minced
- 2 teaspoons olive oil
- 1 cup quinoa, cooked
- ½ cup cherry tomatoes, halved
- 1 carrot, shredded
- 1 roasted red pepper, cubed
- 1 green onion, chopped
- A pinch of salt and black pepper
- 2 teaspoons lemon juice
- 4 eggs, fried

Directions:
Heat up a pan with the olive oil over medium-high heat, add the chard, stir and cook for 1-2 minutes. Add the garlic, tomatoes, carrot, red pepper, onions, salt and pepper, toss and cook for 2 minutes more. Add the quinoa and the lemon juice, toss, cook for 1 minute, divide into bowls, top each bowl with a fried egg and serve for breakfast.
Enjoy!

Nutrition: calories 211, fat 2, fiber 4, carbs 15, protein 6

Veggie Bowls

Preparation time: 10 minutes
Cooking time: 1 hour
Servings: 2

Ingredients:

- 1½ cups black barley
- 4 cups water
- 2 cups blueberries
- 1 fennel bulb, shaved
- 1 bunch watercress
- 1 orange, peeled and cut into segments
- 1 small red onion, sliced
- ¼ cup walnuts
- 1 avocado, peeled, pitted and cubed

For the dressing:

- ½ cup orange juice
- ¼ cup olive oil
- 1 small red onion, chopped
- 2 tablespoons red vinegar
- 1 tablespoon raw honey
- 1 teaspoon bee pollen
- A pinch of salt and black pepper

Directions:

Put the barley in a small pot, add the water and bring to a simmer, Cook for 1 hour, drain and let the mix cool down before putting it in a salad bowl. Add the blueberries, fennel, watercress, orange, 1 red onion, avocado and walnuts and toss. In another bowl, whisk together the orange juice with the oil, onion, vinegar, honey, bee pollen, salt and pepper. Pour over the salad and serve for breakfast.
Enjoy!
Nutrition: calories 216, fat 11, fiber 7, carbs 15, protein 5

Chili Veggie and Quinoa Bowls

Preparation time: 10 minutes
Cooking time: 0 minutes
Servings: 2

Ingredients:

- ½ cup quinoa, cooked
- 1 scallion, chopped
- 1 sweet potato, peeled, cooked and cubed
- 1 bunch broccolini, steamed
- 2 carrots, shredded
- ¼ cup pomegranate seeds
- A handful bean sprouts, soaked for 12 hours, drained

- 1 teaspoon sesame seeds
- 1 tablespoon olive oil
- 2 tablespoons orange juice
- 1 teaspoon coconut aminos
- 1 teaspoon sesame oil
- 1 teaspoon chili paste
- 1 teaspoon white vinegar

Directions:

In a bowl, whisk the sesame oil with the orange juice, aminos, chili paste and vinegar. In a separate salad bowl, mix the scallion with the quinoa, sweet potato, broccolini, carrots, pomegranate seeds, bean sprouts, sesame seeds and olive oil. Add the chili mix and toss the salad together then serve for breakfast.
Enjoy!
Nutrition: calories 171, fat 2, fiber 6, carbs 11, protein 5

Colorful Veggie Mix

Preparation time: 10 minutes
Cooking time: 0 minutes
Servings: 4

Ingredients:

- 1½ cups coconut cream
- ½ cup coconut milk
- 2 tablespoons olive oil
- 2 teaspoons white vinegar
- 1 garlic clove, minced
- 1 teaspoon chopped dill
- ¼ cup chopped parsley
- 1 handful chives, chopped
- 1 jalapeno, chopped
- 1 cup quinoa, cooked
- 1 cup beans sprouts, soaked for 12 hours and drained
- 2 cups cherry tomatoes, halved
- 1½ cups sliced cucumbers
- 2 avocados, peeled, pitted and cubed
- A handful basil, chopped
- 1 tablespoon crushed almonds
- A pinch of salt and black pepper

Directions:

In a salad bowl, mix the quinoa with the bean sprouts, tomatoes, cucumbers, avocados, basil, almonds, salt and pepper. In a separate bowl, whisk the oil with the vinegar, garlic, coconut milk and cream, dill, parsley, chives and jalapeno. Add the dressing to your salad, toss and serve for breakfast.

Enjoy!

Nutrition: calories 199, fat 4, fiber 8, carbs 15, protein 4

Mediterranean Veggie Mix

Preparation time: 10 minutes
Cooking time: 30 minutes
Servings: 4

Ingredients:

- 2 zucchinis, cubed
- 1 eggplant, cubed
- 2 cups quinoa, cooked
- 1 tablespoon olive oil
- ½ teaspoon smoked paprika
- A pinch of chili powder
- 1 tablespoon lemon juice
- A pinch of salt and black pepper
- 1 tablespoon chopped oregano
- 4 cups baby arugula, torn
- ½ cup sesame seeds paste
- 2 tablespoons lemon juice
- 1 teaspoon red wine vinegar
- 1 garlic clove, minced
- 1 teaspoon real maple syrup
- ¾ teaspoon harissa paste
- ½ teaspoon smoked paprika
- ½ teaspoon ground cumin
- ¾ cup water

Directions:

Spread the zucchinis and the eggplant on a lined baking sheet and season with ½ teaspoon smoked paprika, chili powder, salt, pepper, and ½ tablespoon oil. Toss the veggies to coat in the seasoning then bake in the oven at 400 degrees F for 30 minutes. Cool the veggies down, put them in a salad bowl and add the oregano, baby arugula, quinoa, ½ tablespoon oil and lemon juice. Mix together briefly. In another bowl, whisk together the sesame paste with 2 tablespoons lemon juice, vinegar, garlic, maple syrup, harissa paste, ½ teaspoon smoked paprika, cumin and water. Pour the dressing over the salad, toss and serve for breakfast.

Enjoy!

Nutrition: calories 226, fat 5, fiber 7, carbs 16, protein 7

Zucchini and Egg Breakfast Bowl

Preparation time: 10 minutes
Cooking time: 2 hours
Servings: 4

Ingredients:

- 2 zucchinis, cut with a spiralizer
- 1 small avocado, pitted, peeled and chopped
- 2 tablespoons water
- 4 tablespoons olive oil
- 2 sweet potatoes, peeled and cubed
- 2 tablespoons chopped green onion
- 2 garlic cloves, minced
- 2 eggs, whisked
- A pinch of salt and black pepper

Directions:

Heat up a pan with the oil over medium-high heat. Add the green onion and garlic, a pinch of salt and pepper then stir and cook for 2-3 minutes. Transfer the mix to your slow cooker. Add zucchinis, water, potatoes and whisked eggs, toss, cover and cook on High for 2 hours. Divide the mix into bowls, top each with some avocado pieces and serve for breakfast.
Enjoy!

Nutrition: calories 211, fat 2, fiber 5, carbs 16, protein 5

Easy Almond Zucchini Bowl

Preparation time: 10 minutes
Cooking time: 15 minutes
Servings: 2

Ingredients:

- 1 cup egg whites, whisked
- 1½ tablespoons ground flaxseed
- 1 cup almond milk, unsweetened
- 1 banana, peeled and mashed
- 1 small zucchini, grated
- ½ teaspoon ground cinnamon

Directions:

In a small pan, combine the milk with the egg whites, flaxseed, banana, zucchini and cinnamon powder. Bring to a simmer, mixing constantly, over medium heat. Cook for 15 minutes, divide into bowls and serve for breakfast.
Enjoy!

Nutrition: calories 201, fat 6, fiber 9, carbs 14, protein 6

Blueberry and Cashew Mix

Preparation time: 10 minutes
Cooking time: 12 minutes
Servings: 2

Ingredients:

- 2 bananas, peeled and sliced
- ¼ cup cashews
- ¼ cup blueberries
- 1 tablespoon almond butter
- 1/3 cup coconut flakes, unsweetened
- 1 cup coconut milk, unsweetened

Directions:
In a small pot, mix the berries with the coconut flakes, milk, cashews, almond butter and bananas. Mix together and bring to a simmer over medium heat. Cook for 12 minutes, divide into bowls and serve for breakfast.
Enjoy!

Nutrition: calories 370, fat 23, fiber 6, carbs 40, protein 8

Tomato and Olive Salad

Preparation time: 10 minutes
Cooking time: 0 minutes
Servings: 4

Ingredients:

- 2 cups baby spinach, torn
- 2 cups cherry tomatoes, halved
- 4 tablespoons chopped red onion
- 1 cup chopped cucumber
- 1 cup kalamata olives, pitted and sliced
- 1 tablespoon chopped dill
- 3 tablespoons lemon juice
- A pinch of salt and black pepper
- 2 tablespoons olive oil

Directions:
In a salad bowl, toss the spinach with the tomatoes, onion, cucumber, olives, dill, lemon juice, salt, pepper and oil. Serve for breakfast.
Enjoy!

Nutrition: calories 171, fat 2, fiber 5, carbs 11, protein 5

Sweet Potato Hash

Preparation time: 10 minutes
Cooking time: 15 minutes
Servings: 4

Ingredients:

- 1 sweet potato, peeled and cubed
- 1 celery root, peeled and cubed
- 1 cup coconut milk
- 2 tablespoons olive oil
- 1 small yellow onion, chopped
- 1 teaspoon smoked paprika
- 4 garlic cloves, minced
- 2 tablespoons parsley, chopped
- A pinch of salt and black pepper

Directions:

Heat up a pan with the oil over medium-high heat. Add the celery root and the sweet potato, toss and cook for 5 minutes. Add the onion, garlic, salt, pepper, parsley and paprika then toss and cook for 8 minutes more. Add the coconut milk, mix and cook for 1-2 minutes. Divide everything into bowls and serve for breakfast.
Enjoy!

Nutrition: calories 188, fat 2, fiber 8, carbs 10, protein 4

Avocado Omelet

Preparation time: 10 minutes
Cooking time: 10 minutes
Servings: 2

Ingredients:

- 4 eggs, whisked
- 2 avocados, pitted, peeled and cubed
- A pinch of salt and black pepper
- Juice of ½ lemon
- 1 tablespoon chopped parsley
- 1 tablespoon olive oil

Directions:

In a bowl, mix the eggs with the avocados, salt, pepper, lemon juice and parsley. Heat up a pan with the oil over medium-high heat then add the avocado and egg mix, spread into the pan and cook for 4 minutes on each side. Divide between plates and serve for breakfast.
Enjoy!

Nutrition: calories 201, fat 2, fiber 5, carbs 11, protein 5

Coconut Porridge

Preparation time: 10 minutes
Cooking time: 15 minutes
Servings: 2

Ingredients:
- 2 cups coconut milk, unsweetened
- 3 tablespoons almond flour
- ½ cup coconut flakes, unsweetened
- 2 tablespoons ground flax meal
- 1 teaspoon vanilla extract
- 2 teaspoons ground cinnamon

Directions:
In a small pot, mix the coconut milk with the almond flour, coconut flakes, flax meal, vanilla and cinnamon. Stir and bring to a simmer over medium heat for 15 minutes. Divide into bowls and serve for breakfast.
Enjoy!

Nutrition: calories 287, fat 5, fiber 7, carbs 13, protein 5

Broccoli and Squash Mix

Preparation time: 10 minutes
Cooking time: 15 minutes
Servings: 4

Ingredients:
- 4 cups spaghetti squash, peeled, cooked and flesh scrapped out
- 1½ cups broccoli florets
- 1 tablespoon olive oil
- 1 cup coconut milk, unsweetened
- 1 egg, whisked
- 1 teaspoon garlic powder
- A pinch of salt and black pepper

Directions:
Heat up a pan with the oil over medium-high heat, add the spaghetti squash and the broccoli. Stir and cook for 5-6 minutes. Add the garlic powder, salt, pepper, garlic powder and the egg. Stir and cook for 5 minutes more. Add the coconut milk, mix and cook for about 5 minutes more then divide into bowls and serve for breakfast.
Enjoy!

Nutrition: calories 207, fat 5, fiber 8, carbs 14, protein 7

Greens and Berries Mix

Preparation time: 10 minutes
Cooking time: 0 minutes
Servings: 2

Ingredients:
- ½ cup spinach, torn
- ½ cup kale, torn
- 1 cup strawberries, halved
- 1 cup blueberries
- 1 banana, peeled and chopped
- 6 mint leaves, chopped

Directions:
In a bowl, mix the spinach with the kale, strawberries, blueberries, banana and mint. Serve for breakfast.
Enjoy!

Nutrition: calories 198, fat 4, fiber 2, carbs 8, protein 6

Veggie and Eggs

Preparation time: 10 minutes
Cooking time: 15 minutes
Servings: 6

Ingredients:
- 1 red bell pepper, chopped
- 4 cherry tomatoes, chopped
- 3 spring onions, chopped
- A handful kale, torn
- 1 tablespoon olive oil
- 6 eggs
- A pinch of salt and black pepper
- A pinch of curry powder

Directions:
Heat up a pan with the oil over medium-high heat, add the onions, stir and cook for 1-2 minutes. Add the bell pepper, the tomatoes, the kale, salt, pepper and the curry powder, stir and cook for 4-5 minutes. Crack the eggs into the pan and mix well. Cook until the eggs are done, divide between plates and serve for breakfast.
Enjoy!

Nutrition: calories 106, fat 8, fiber 1, carbs 4, protein 7

Coconut Pear Bowl

Preparation time: 10 minutes
Cooking time: 15 minutes
Servings: 4

Ingredients:

- 2 cups coconut milk, unsweetened
- 1/3 cup coconut flakes, unsweetened
- ½ teaspoon vanilla extract
- 3 pears, peeled, cored and cubed

Directions:
Put the milk in a small pot, add the coconut, vanilla and pears. Stir and bring to a simmer over medium heat, cook for 15 minutes, divide into bowls and serve.
Enjoy!

Nutrition: calories 172, fat 5, fiber 7, carbs 8, protein 4

Blackberry and Strawberry Salad

Preparation time: 5 minutes
Cooking time: 0 minutes
Servings: 1

Ingredients:

- ¼ cup sliced almonds
- ¼ cup blackberries
- ¼ cup strawberries, halved
- 1 banana, peeled and sliced
- A pinch of ground cinnamon

Directions:
In a bowl, mix the blackberries with strawberries, cinnamon, banana and almonds. Serve for breakfast.
Enjoy!

Nutrition: calories 90, fat 0.3, fiber 1, carbs 0, protein 5

Breakfast Kale Frittata

Preparation time: 10 minutes
Cooking time: 30 minutes
Servings: 4

Ingredients:

- 6 kale stalks, chopped
- 1 small sweet onion, chopped
- 1 small broccoli head, florets separated
- 2 garlic cloves, minced
- Salt and black pepper to the taste
- 4 eggs
- 1 tablespoon olive oil

Directions:
Heat up a pan with the oil over medium-high heat, add the onion, stir and cook for 4-5 minutes. Add the garlic, broccoli and kale, toss and cook for 5 minutes more. Add the eggs, salt and pepper and mix. Place in the oven and bake at 380 degrees F for 20 minutes. Slice and serve for breakfast.
Enjoy!

Nutrition: calories 214, fat 7, fiber 2, carbs 12, protein 8

Cranberry Granola Bars

Preparation time: 2 hours
Cooking time: 0 minutes
Servings: 4

Ingredients:

- 2 cups walnuts, toasted
- 1 cup dates, pitted
- 3 tablespoons water
- ¾ cup cranberries, dried, no added sugar
- 2 cups desiccated coconut, unsweetened

Directions:
In your food processor, mix dates with coconut, cranberries, water and walnuts. Pulse really well then spread the mix into a lined baking dish. Press well into the dish and keep in the fridge for 2 hours then cut into bars and serve.
Enjoy!

Nutrition: calories 476, fat 40, fiber 9, carbs 33, protein 6

Spinach and Berry Smoothie

Preparation time: 10 minutes
Cooking time: 0 minutes
Servings: 2

Ingredients:
- 1 cup blackberries
- 1 avocado, pitted, peeled and chopped
- 1 banana, peeled and roughly chopped
- 1 cup baby spinach
- 1 tablespoon hemp seeds
- 1 cup water
- ½ cup almond milk, unsweetened

Directions:
In your blender, mix the berries with the avocado, banana, spinach, hemp seeds, water and almond milk. Pulse well, divide into 2 glasses and serve for breakfast.
Enjoy!

Nutrition: calories 160, fat 3, fiber 4, carbs 6, protein 3

Zucchini Breakfast Salad

Preparation time: 10 minutes
Cooking time: 0 minutes
Servings: 4

Ingredients:
- 2 zucchinis, spiralized
- 1 cup beets, baked, peeled and grated
- ½ bunch kale, chopped
- 2 tablespoons olive oil

For the tahini sauce:
- 1 tablespoon maple syrup
- Juice of 1 lime
- ¼ inch fresh ginger, grated
- 1/3 cup sesame seed paste

Directions:
In a salad bowl, mix the zucchinis with the beets, kale and oil. In another small bowl, whisk the maple syrup with lime juice, ginger and sesame paste. Pour the dressing over the salad, toss and serve it for breakfast.
Enjoy!

Nutrition: calories 183, fat 3, fiber 2, carbs 7, protein 9

Quinoa and Spinach Breakfast Salad

Preparation time: 10 minutes
Cooking time: 0 minutes
Servings: 2

Ingredients:

- 16 ounces quinoa, cooked
- 1 handful raisins
- 1 handful baby spinach leaves
- 1 tablespoon maple syrup
- ½ tablespoon lemon juice
- 4 tablespoons olive oil
- 1 teaspoon ground cumin
- A pinch of sea salt and black pepper
- ½ teaspoon chili flakes

Directions:

In a bowl, mix the quinoa with the spinach, raisins, cumin, salt and pepper and toss. Add the maple syrup, lemon juice, oil and chili flakes and toss then serve for breakfast.
Enjoy!

Nutrition: calories 170, fat 3, fiber 6, carbs 8, protein 5

Carrots Breakfast Mix

Preparation time: 10 minutes
Cooking time: 0 minutes
Servings: 4

Ingredients:

- 1½ tablespoon maple syrup
- 1 teaspoon olive oil
- 1 tablespoon chopped walnuts
- 1 onion, chopped
- 4 cups shredded carrots
- 1 tablespoon curry powder
- ¼ teaspoon ground turmeric
- Black pepper to the taste
- 2 tablespoons sesame seed paste
- ¼ cup lemon juice
- ½ cup chopped parsley

Directions:

In a salad bowl, mix together the onion with the carrots, turmeric, curry powder, black pepper, lemon juice and parsley. Add the maple syrup, oil, walnuts and sesame seed paste. Toss well and serve for breakfast.
Enjoy!

Nutrition: calories 150, fat 3, fiber 2, carbs 6, protein 8

Italian Breakfast Salad

Preparation time: 10 minutes
Cooking time: 0 minutes
Servings: 4

Ingredients:

- 1 handful kalamata olives, pitted and sliced
- 1 cup cherry tomatoes, halved
- 1½ cucumbers, sliced
- 1 red onion, chopped
- 2 tablespoons chopped oregano
- 1 tablespoon chopped mint

For the salad dressing:

- 2 tablespoons balsamic vinegar
- ¼ cup olive oil
- 1 garlic clove, minced
- 2 teaspoons dried Italian herbs
- A pinch of salt and black pepper

Directions:

In a salad bowl, toss together the olives with the tomatoes, cucumbers, onion, mint and oregano. In a smaller bowl, whisk the vinegar with the oil, garlic, Italian herbs, salt and pepper. Pour the dressing over the salad, toss and serve for breakfast.
Enjoy!

Nutrition: calories 191, fat 10, fiber 3, carbs 13, protein 1

Zucchini and Sprout Breakfast Mix

Preparation time: 10 minutes
Cooking time: 0 minutes
Servings: 4

Ingredients:

- 2 zucchinis, spiralized
- 2 cups bean sprouts
- 4 green onions, chopped
- 1 red bell pepper, chopped
- Juice of 1 lime

- 1 tablespoon olive oil
- ½ cup chopped cilantro
- ¾ cup almonds chopped
- A pinch of salt and black pepper

Directions:

In a salad bowl, toss together the zucchinis with the bean sprouts, green onions, bell pepper, cilantro, almonds, salt, pepper, limejuice and oil. Serve for breakfast.

Nutrition: calories 140, fat 4, fiber 2, carbs 7, protein 8

Breakfast Corn Salad

Preparation time: 10 minutes
Cooking time: 0 minutes
Servings: 4

Ingredients:

- 2 avocados, pitted, peeled and cubed
- 1-pint mixed cherry tomatoes, halved
- 2 cups fresh corn kernels
- 1 red onion, chopped

For the salad dressing:
- 2 tablespoons olive oil
- 1 tablespoon lime juice
- ½ teaspoon grated lime zest
- A pinch of salt and black pepper
- ¼ cup chopped cilantro

Directions:
In a salad bowl, mix the avocados with the tomatoes, corn and onion. Add the oil, lime juice, lime zest, salt, pepper and the cilantro, toss and serve for breakfast.

Nutrition: calories 140, fat 3, fiber 2, carbs 6, protein 9

Simple Basil Tomato Mix

Preparation time: 10 minutes
Cooking time: 0 minutes
Servings: 6

Ingredients:

- ½ cup extra-virgin olive oil
- 1 cucumber, chopped
- 2 pints colored cherry tomatoes, halved
- Salt and black pepper to the taste

- 1 red onion, chopped
- 3 tablespoons red vinegar
- 1 garlic clove, minced
- 1 bunch basil, roughly chopped

Directions:
In a salad bowl, toss together the cucumber with the tomatoes, onion, salt, pepper, oil, vinegar, basil and garlic. Serve for breakfast.
Enjoy!

Nutrition: calories 100, fat 1, fiber 2, carbs 2, protein 6

Cucumber and Avocado Salad

Preparation time: 10 minutes
Cooking time: 0 minutes
Servings: 4

Ingredients:

- 1 pound cucumbers, chopped
- 2 avocados, pitted and chopped
- 1 small red onion, thinly sliced
- 2 tablespoons olive oil
- 2 tablespoons lemon juice
- ¼ cup chopped parsley
- A pinch of salt and black pepper

Directions:
In a salad bowl, mix together the cucumbers with the avocados, onion, oil, lemon juice, parsley, salt and pepper. Serve for breakfast.
Enjoy!

Nutrition: calories 120, fat 2, fiber 2, carbs 3, protein 4

Watermelon Salad

Preparation time: 10 minutes
Cooking time: 0 minutes
Servings:2

Ingredients:

- ½ teaspoon agave nectar
- 2 tablespoons lemon juice
- 1 tablespoon extra-virgin olive oil
- 1 jalapeno, seeded and chopped
- 12 ounces watermelon, chopped
- 1 red onion, thinly sliced
- ½ cup chopped basil leaves
- 2 cups baby arugula

Directions:
In a bowl, toss together the watermelon with the jalapeno, onion, basil, arugula, oil, agave nectar, lemon juice and oil. Serve for breakfast.

Nutrition: calories 128, fat 8, fiber 2, carbs 16, protein 2

Lunch Recipes

Carrot and Turmeric Soup

Preparation time: 10 minutes
Cooking time: 15 minutes
Servings: 2

Ingredients:

- 1 parsnip, chopped
- 4 carrots, chopped
- 1 yellow onion, chopped
- 4 garlic cloves, minced
- 2 teaspoons coconut oil, melted
- 1 teaspoon ground turmeric
- 3 cups veggie stock
- 1 teaspoon fresh grated ginger
- Juice of ½ lemon
- A pinch of cayenne pepper
- 1 tablespoon chopped parsley

Directions:

Spread the carrots, the parsnip, the garlic and onion on a lined baking sheet and drizzle with the olive oil. Season with turmeric and cayenne then toss and bake in the oven for 15 minutes at 350 degrees F. Once cooked transfer to a blender and puree. Heat up the stock over medium heat, add lemon juice and ginger. Stir the stock mix then transfer to the blender as well and pulse the soup. Ladle into bowls, sprinkle the parsley on top and serve for lunch.
Enjoy!

Nutrition: calories 200, fat 4, fiber 4, carbs 11, protein 6

Easy Lentil Soup

Preparation time: 10 minutes
Cooking time: 25 minutes
Servings: 7

Ingredients:

- 2 cups chopped yellow onion
- 1½ tablespoons olive oil
- 2 garlic cloves, minced
- 1½ teaspoon ground cumin
- 2 teaspoons ground turmeric
- ½ teaspoon ground cinnamon
- ¼ teaspoon ground cardamom
- 15 ounces canned tomatoes, chopped
- 14 ounces coconut milk, unsweetened
- ¾ cup red lentils, rinsed
- 3 cups veggie stock
- A pinch of salt and black pepper
- 6 ounces baby spinach
- 2 teaspoons lime juice

Directions:

Heat up a pot with the olive oil over medium heat, add the garlic and the onion, stir and sauté for 5 minutes. Add cardamom, cinnamon, cumin and turmeric, stir and cook for 1 minute. Add tomatoes, coconut milk, lentils, stock, salt and pepper. Stir the soup, bring it to a simmer and cook for 17 minutes. Add the spinach and lime juice, mix and ladle the soup into bowls and serve.
Enjoy!

Nutrition: calories 211, fat 4, fiber 4, carbs 14, protein 6

Quinoa Lunch Bowls

Preparation time: 10 minutes
Cooking time: 30 minutes
Servings: 4

Ingredients:

- 15 ounces canned chickpeas, drained
- 8 small potatoes, cubed
- 1 teaspoon sweet paprika
- 2 teaspoons ground turmeric
- 1 tablespoon coconut oil, melted
- ¼ cup quinoa
- A pinch of salt and black pepper
- ½ tablespoon olive oil
- 2 kale leaves, torn
- 1 avocado, pitted, peeled and sliced

Directions:
Spread the potatoes on a lined baking sheet and drizzle the coconut oil over them. Sprinkle half of the turmeric, season with salt and pepper and place in the oven. Bake at 350 degrees F for 5 minutes then set aside for a few minutes to cool.In aseparate bowl, mix the chickpeas with the paprika and spread them on another baking sheet. Roast in the oven at 350 degrees F for 20 minutes.In another salad bowl, mix roasted potatoes with the chickpeas, the remaining turmeric, olive oil, salt, pepper, quinoa, kale and avocado. Mix everything together well and serve for lunch.
Enjoy!

Nutrition: calories 300, fat 4, fiber 7, carbs 15, protein 7

Salmon and Broccoli

Preparation time: 10 minutes
Cooking time: 15 minutes
Servings: 4

Ingredients:

- 1 broccoli head, florets separated
- 1½ pound salmon fillets, boneless
- 3 tablespoons avocado oil
- 2 garlic cloves, minced
- A pinch of salt and black pepper
- Juice of ½ lemon

Directions:
Spread the broccoli on a lined baking sheet, add the salmon, oil, garlic, salt, pepper and the lemon juice. Mix gently to coat the salmon and broccoli with the seasonings then place in the oven and bake at 450 degrees F for 15 minutes. Divide everything between plates and serve.
Enjoy!

Nutrition: calories 294, fat 13, fiber 6, carbs 13, protein 26

Italian Chicken

Preparation time: 10 minutes
Cooking time: 1 hour
Servings: 6

Ingredients:

- 6 chicken thighs, boneless and skinless
- 2 sweet potatoes, cut into wedges
- 2 tablespoons olive oil
- 1 tablespoon lemon juice
- 1 cup chopped parsley
- 2 tablespoons Italian seasoning

Directions:
Spread the chicken on a lined baking sheet, add the potatoes, oil, lemon juice, parsley and seasoning. Toss everything on the tray to mix well then bake in the oven at 350 degrees F for 1 hour. Divide everything between plates and serve.
Enjoy!

Nutrition: calories 241, fat 7, fiber 8, carbs 11, protein 7

Balsamic Salmon

Preparation time: 10 minutes
Cooking time: 20 minutes
Servings: 4

Ingredients:

- 4 salmon fillets, boneless and skin-on
- 15 ounces baby potatoes, halved
- 1 bunch asparagus, halved and trimmed
- 15 ounces Brussels sprouts, halved
- 1 small red onion, cubed
- 2 tablespoons olive oil
- 1 cup cherry tomatoes, halved
- 3 tablespoons balsamic vinegar
- 1 tablespoon mustard
- 1 garlic clove, minced
- 1 teaspoon chopped thyme
- A pinch of salt and black pepper

Directions:
Spread the baby potatoes on a lined baking sheet. Add the asparagus, Brussels sprouts, onion, tomatoes, vinegar, garlic, salt, pepper, thyme and oil. Toss everything on the tray together then place in the oven and bake at 450 degrees F for 10 minutes. Remove the tray from the oven and add the salmon. Season with salt and pepper then return to the oven for 10 minutes more, divide everything between plates and serve for lunch.
Enjoy!

Nutrition: calories 266, fat 11, fiber 6, carbs 14, protein 9

Shrimp and Bok Choy Soup

Preparation time: 10 minutes
Cooking time: 30 minutes
Servings: 4

Ingredients:

- 1 yellow onion, chopped
- 1 tablespoon olive oil
- 6 garlic cloves, minced
- A pinch of salt and black pepper
- 1 teaspoon ground turmeric
- 6 cups chicken stock
- 1 pound mushrooms, sliced
- 2 carrots, sliced
- 6 bok choy heads, torn
- 1 pound shrimp, deveined and peeled

Directions:

Heat up a pot with the oil over medium heat, add the garlic and the onions, stir and sauté for 5 minutes. Add the stock, carrots, mushrooms, salt, pepper and the turmeric. Bring to a simmer, stir and cook for 20 minutes. Add the bok choy and the shrimp, stir and cook for 5 minutes more then ladle everything into bowls and serve.
Enjoy!

Nutrition: calories 261, fat 7, fiber 8, carbs 16, protein 11

Chickpea Cakes

Preparation time: 10 minutes
Cooking time: 10 minutes
Servings: 4

Ingredients:

- 2 garlic cloves, peeled
- 1 yellow onion, peeled and chopped
- 1½ cups canned chickpeas, drained and rinsed
- ¼ cup parsley leaves
- 2 tablespoons coconut flour
- 2 tablespoons chickpeas flour
- 1 teaspoon ground turmeric
- A pinch of salt and black pepper
- A pinch of cayenne pepper
- 3 tablespoons grapeseed oil

Directions:

In a blender, mix the garlic with the onion, chickpeas, parsley, coconut flour, turmeric, salt, pepper and cayenne. Pulse well and shape medium cakes out of this mix. Dredge them in the chickpea flour then directly into a preheated pan with the oil over medium heat. Cook for 5 minutes on each side and serve them for lunch.
Enjoy!

Nutrition: calories 261, fat 4, fiber 7, carbs 15, protein 7

Simple Roasted Sweet Potatoes and Sauce

Preparation time: 10 minutes
Cooking time: 45 minutes
Servings: 4

Ingredients:

- 2 sweet potatoes, peeled and cubed
- 2½ tablespoons olive oil
- A pinch of salt and black pepper
- 1 garlic clove, minced
- 1 avocado, pitted, peeled and halved
- Juice of 1 lime
- 4 tablespoons water

Directions:

Spread the potatoes on a lined baking sheet and drizzle with ½ tablespoon oil. Season with salt and pepper, place in the oven and bake at 400 degrees F for 45 minutes. Meanwhile, in your blender, mix the avocado with garlic, lime juice, water, the rest of the oil, salt and pepper. Pulse the blender well and transfer the mix to a bowl. Serve your roasted potatoes with the avocado sauce on the side.
Enjoy!

Nutrition: calories 222, fat 6, fiber 7, carbs 15, protein 7

Lemony Lentil Soup

Preparation time: 10 minutes
Cooking time: 1 hour and 20 minutes
Servings: 6

Ingredients:

- 1½ cups carrots, sliced
- 1 tablespoon olive oil
- 1 yellow onion, chopped
- 1½ cups chopped celery
- 3 garlic cloves, minced
- A pinch of salt and black pepper
- 4 teaspoons fresh grated ginger
- 32 ounces veggie stock
- 2 teaspoons ground turmeric
- 2 cups green lentils, rinsed
- Juice of 3 small lemons
- Zest of ½ lemon, grated

Directions:

Heat up a pot with the oil over medium heat and add the celery, carrots, onion, a pinch of salt and pepper. Mix together and sauté for 5 minutes. Add the ginger and the garlic, stir and cook for 1 minute more. Add the lentils, stock and turmeric. Stir, reduce heat to low, cover the pot and cook for 45 minutes. Add lemon juice and lemon zest, stir and cook the soup for 30 minutes more. Ladle into bowls and serve.
Enjoy!

Nutrition: calories 271, fat 8, fiber 11, carbs 16, protein 8

Veggie and Egg Burrito Bowls

Preparation time: 10 minutes
Cooking time: 8 minutes
Servings: 1

Ingredients:

- ¼ cup spinach leaves, torn
- 1 tablespoon black olives, pitted and chopped
- 1 tablespoon chopped red bell pepper
- 1 teaspoon olive oil
- 3 cherry tomatoes, halved
- 2 eggs, whisked
- 1 tablespoon chopped parsley
- Avocado mayonnaise for serving

Directions:
Heat up a pan with the olive oil over medium-high heat. Add olives, bell pepper, tomatoes and spinach, stir and cook for 3 minutes. Add the eggs, stir and cook until everything is done (about 1-2 minutes). Divide into bowls, sprinkle with parsley, top with avocado mayonnaise and serve. Enjoy!

Nutrition: calories 217, fat 18, fiber 2, carbs 6, protein 14

Turkey Burgers

Preparation time: 10 minutes
Cooking time: 10 minutes
Servings: 4

Ingredients:

- 1 pound turkey meat, ground
- 1 shallot, minced
- 1 tablespoon olive oil
- 1 small jalapeno pepper, minced
- 2 teaspoons lime juice
- Zest of 1 lime, grated
- Salt and black pepper to the taste
- 1 teaspoon turmeric powder

Directions:
In a bowl, mix the turkey meat with shallot, jalapeno, lime juice, lime zest, salt, pepper and turmeric stir well and shape medium burgers out of this mix. Heat up a pan with the oil over medium-high heat, add the turkey burgers, cook them for about 5 minutes on each side, divide between plates and serve for lunch.
Enjoy!

Nutrition: calories 200, fat 12, fiber 5, carbs 12, protein 7

Turkey Soup

Preparation time: 10 minutes
Cooking time: 40 minutes
Servings: 4

Ingredients:

- 4 shallots, chopped
- 3 carrots, chopped
- 1 pound ground turkey
- Salt and black pepper to the taste
- 1 red bell pepper, chopped
- 5 cups vegetable stock
- 1½ cups cauliflower florets, chopped
- 4 cups kale, chopped
- 2 tablespoons coconut oil, melted
- 15 ounces canned tomatoes, chopped

Directions:
Heat up a pot with the oil over medium-high heat. Add shallots, cauliflower, bell pepper and carrots, stir and cook for 10 minutes. Add ground turkey, stir and cook for 8 more minutes. Add tomatoes, salt, pepper, kale and stock. Stir, bring to a boil, cover, cook for 15 minutes then ladle into bowls and serve
Enjoy!

Nutrition: calories 210, fat 1, fiber 5, carbs 14, protein 6

Poached Cod

Preparation time: 10 minutes
Cooking time: 25 minutes
Servings: 4

Ingredients:

- 4 cod fillets, skinless
- 3 garlic cloves, minced
- 1 yellow onion, chopped
- Salt and black pepper to the taste
- 2 tablespoons olive oil
- 2 tablespoons chopped tarragon
- ¼ cup chopped parsley
- Juice of 1 lemon
- 1 lemon, sliced
- 1 tablespoon chopped thyme
- 4 cups water

Directions:
Heat up a pan with the oil over medium-high heat, Add onion and garlic, stir and cook for 3 minutes. Add salt, pepper, tarragon, parsley, thyme, water, lemon juice and lemon slices, stir and bring to a gentle boil. Add cod, cook for 15 minutes, drain and serve with a side salad.
Enjoy!

Nutrition: calories 173, fat 3, fiber 4, carbs 9, protein 12

Chicken and Kale Soup

Preparation time: 10 minutes
Cooking time: 15 minutes
Servings: 6

Ingredients:
- 1 bunch kale, chopped
- Salt and black pepper to the taste
- 2 quarts vegetable stock
- 1 cup cooked shredded chicken
- 3 carrots, chopped
- 1 tablespoon chopped parsley
- 1 cup white mushrooms, sliced

Directions:
Heat up a pot with the stock over medium heat, add carrots, mushrooms, chicken, kale, salt and pepper. Stir the soup, bring to a simmer and cook for 15 minutes. Ladle into bowls and serve for lunch.
Enjoy!

Nutrition: calories 210, fat 7, fiber 2, carbs 10, protein 8

Cod and Fennel

Preparation time: 10 minutes
Cooking time: 15 minutes
Servings: 4

Ingredients:
- 4 cod fillets, boneless
- Salt and black pepper to the taste
- Juice of ½ lemon
- 2 fennel bulbs, sliced
- 1 tablespoon coconut oil, melted
- 1 tablespoon olive oil

Directions:
Heat up a pan with the coconut oil over medium-high heat. Add fennel slices, season with salt and pepper, mix, cover, cook for 10 minutes and divide between plates. Heat up a pan with the olive oil over medium-high heat, add fish fillets and season with salt and pepper. Cook for 3 minutes, flip and cook for 2 more minutes. Serve next to the fennel and drizzle the lemon juice all over the plate before serving.
Enjoy!

Nutrition: calories 200, fat 2, fiber 4, carbs 10, protein 8

Broccoli Soup

Preparation time: 10 minutes
Cooking time: 25 minutes
Servings: 4

Ingredients:

- 4 leeks, chopped
- 2 tablespoons olive oil
- 1 yellow onion, chopped
- Salt and black pepper to the taste
- 1½ pounds broccoli florets, chopped
- 3 shallots, chopped
- ¼ apple, chopped
- 1-quart vegetable stock
- ½ teaspoon ground turmeric
- 1 teaspoon ground curry
- 1 cup coconut milk, unsweetened

Directions:

Heat up a soup pot with the oil over medium heat and add onions, leeks and shallots. Stir and cook for 6 minutes. Add apple, broccoli and stock, turmeric, curry powder, salt and pepper and stir. Cook over medium heat for 20 minutes. Transfer mix to a blender, add coconut milk, pulse well, divide into bowls and serve.
Enjoy!

Nutrition: calories 210, fat 8, fiber 6, carbs 10, protein 7

Cauliflower Cream

Preparation time: 10 minutes
Cooking time: 50 minutes
Servings: 4

Ingredients:

- 3 pounds cauliflower, florets separated
- 1 yellow onion, chopped
- 1 tablespoon coconut oil
- A pinch of salt and black pepper
- 2 garlic cloves, minced
- 2 carrots, chopped
- 3 cups vegetable soup
- ½ cup coconut milk, unsweetened
- A pinch of nutmeg
- A pinch of cayenne pepper
- A handful parsley, chopped

Directions:

Heat up a pot with the oil over medium-high heat, add carrots, onion and garlic then stir and cook for 5 minutes. Add cauliflower and stock, stir, bring to a boil, reduce heat, cover, cook for 45 minutes. Transfer the soup to a blender, add the coconut milk, salt and pepper, pulse well, divide into bowls, sprinkle nutmeg, cayenne and parsley on top and serve.
Enjoy!

Nutrition: calories 210, fat 2, fiber 5, carbs 10, protein 7

Chicken Casserole

Preparation time: 10 minutes
Cooking time: 50 minutes
Servings: 4

Ingredients:

- 4 cups broccoli florets
- 1 yellow onion, chopped
- 2 tablespoons olive oil
- Salt and black pepper to the taste
- 8 ounces mushrooms, sliced
- 3 cups chicken, cooked and shredded
- 1 cup chicken stock
- ½ teaspoon ground nutmeg
- 2 eggs

Directions:
Heat up a pan with the oil over medium heat, add onions, mushrooms, salt and pepper, stir, cook for 10 minutes. Pour into a baking dish and top with the chicken and the broccoli. In a bowl, mix stock, eggs, nutmeg, salt and pepper. Stir well, spread over the chicken mix and cook at 350 degrees F for 40 minutes. Divide between plates and serve.
Enjoy!

Nutrition: calories 318, fat 18, fiber 3, carbs 5, protein 33

Chicken Salad

Preparation time: 10 minutes
Cooking time: 10 minutes
Servings: 4

Ingredients:

- 2 sweet potatoes, baked
- A drizzle of olive oil
- 1 yellow onion, chopped
- 12 ounces mushrooms, chopped
- 2 garlic cloves, minced
- ½ teaspoon dried thyme
- 3 cups chicken, already cooked and shredded
- 2 cups baby spinach
- A pinch of salt and cayenne pepper
- A splash of balsamic vinegar

Directions:
Cut potatoes in half lengthwise, scoop out the flesh, chop it and put in a bowl. Heat up a pan with the oil over medium-high heat. Add onion, potato flesh, garlic, mushrooms, thyme, chicken, salt and cayenne pepper, toss, cook for 10 minutes, take off heat and transfer to the bowl with the sweet potato flesh. Add the spinach and the vinegar, toss and serve.
Enjoy!

Nutrition: calories 260, fat 2, fiber 8, carbs 17, protein 11

Italian Zucchini Mix

Preparation time: 10 minutes
Cooking time: 20 minutes
Servings: 4

Ingredients:

- ¼ cup olive oil
- 2 zucchinis, cut into small rounds
- 1 red bell pepper, cut into thin strips
- 1 yellow onion, cut into medium wedges
- 1 eggplant, cubed
- A pinch of ground turmeric
- A pinch of salt and black pepper
- 1 tablespoons capers
- 10 cherry tomatoes, halved
- 2 tablespoons pine nuts
- 1 tablespoons raisins
- 1 bunch basil , chopped

Directions:
Heat up a pan with the oil over medium-high heat, add the onion, salt, pepper and turmeric, mix and cook for 5 minutes. Add the zucchini, bell pepper and eggplant, mix and cook for 5 minutes more. Add the capers, tomatoes, pine nuts and raisins, mix and cook for 10 minutes over medium heat. Add the basil, stir, cook for another minute more. Divide into bowls and serve for lunch. Enjoy!

Nutrition: calories 162, fat 3, fiber 4, carbs 12, protein 7

Cauliflower Stew

Preparation time: 10 minutes
Cooking time: 35 minutes
Servings: 2

Ingredients:

- ½ teaspoon olive oil
- 1 small cauliflower head, florets separated
- ½ teaspoon cumin seeds
- ½ cup red onion, chopped
- 2 tomatoes, chopped
- 1 teaspoon fresh grated ginger
- 4 garlic cloves, minced
- 1 teaspoon ground coriander
- ½ teaspoon ground turmeric
- A pinch of cayenne pepper
- ½ teaspoon garam masala
- 2 cups vegetable stock
- A pinch of salt and black pepper
- 1 teaspoon lemon juice

Directions:
In your blender, add the tomatoes with garlic, onions, ginger, salt, pepper, garam masala, cayenne, coriander and turmeric and pulse really well. Heat up a pot with the oil over medium heat, add the tomato mix, stir and sauté for 15 minutes. Add cauliflower, stock, salt, pepper, lemon juice and cumin, stir, cover and simmer over medium heat for 20 minutes. Divide into bowls and serve.
Enjoy!

Nutrition: calories 200, fat 6, fiber 7, carbs 10, protein 8

Green Bean Lunch Mix

Preparation time: 10 minutes
Cooking time: 25 minutes
Servings: 4

Ingredients:

- 2 tablespoons olive oil
- 2 carrots, chopped
- 1 yellow onion, chopped
- 1 sweet potato, cubed
- 14 ounces green beans
- 2 garlic cloves, minced
- 14 ounces canned tomatoes, chopped
- 1 cup corn
- 5 cups water
- A pinch of salt and black pepper
- 1 tablespoon chopped cilantro

Directions:
Heat up a pan with the oil over medium heat, add onion, stir and cook for 5 minutes. Add carrots, sweet potato, green beans, garlic, tomatoes, corn, salt, pepper and water, stir, cover and cook over medium heat for 20 minutes. Add the cilantro, stir, divide into bowls and serve. Enjoy!

Nutrition: calories 201, fat 5, fiber 5, carbs 8, protein 11

Chickpea Stew

Preparation time: 10 minutes
Cooking time: 50 minutes
Servings: 4

Ingredients:

- 1 teaspoon olive oil
- 1 cup chickpeas, soaked for 4 hours and drained
- 4 garlic cloves, minced
- 1 small yellow onion, chopped
- 1 green chili pepper, chopped
- 1-inch fresh ginger, grated
- 1 teaspoon ground coriander
- ½ teaspoon ground cumin
- ½ teaspoon sweet paprika
- 2 tomatoes, chopped
- 1½ cups water
- A pinch of salt and black pepper
- 3 cups spinach leaves
- 1 tablespoon lemon juice
- 1 cup coconut milk, unsweetened

Directions:
Heat up a pot with the oil over medium heat, add garlic, ginger, chili and onion. Stir and cook for 5 minutes. Add tomatoes, cumin, paprika, coriander, chickpeas, water, salt and pepper to the pot. Stir, bring to a simmer and cook for 45 minutes. Add spinach, lemon juice and coconut milk, stir, and cook for 10 minutes more. Divide into bowls and serve.
Enjoy!

Nutrition: calories 250, fat 7, fiber 6, carbs 9, protein 12

Eggplant Stew

Preparation time: 10 minutes
Cooking time: 15 minutes
Servings: 3

Ingredients:

- ½ teaspoon cumin seeds
- 1 tablespoon coriander seeds
- ½ teaspoon mustard seeds
- 5 eggplants, cubed
- 2 tablespoon coconut, shredded, unsweetened
- 1 teaspoon fresh grated ginger
- 2 garlic cloves, minced
- 1 green chili pepper, chopped
- A pinch of cayenne pepper
- A pinch of ground cinnamon
- ½ teaspoon ground cardamom
- ½ teaspoon ground turmeric
- A pinch of salt and black pepper
- 1 teaspoon lime juice
- 1 cup vegetable stock
- 1 tablespoon chopped parsley

Directions:

Heat up a pan over medium-high heat and add the cumin, coriander, mustard seeds, coconut, ginger, garlic, chili pepper, cayenne, cinnamon, cardamom, turmeric, salt and pepper. Stir and cook for 5-6 minutes. Transfer to a food processor and pulse. Transfer to a pot and heat up over medium heat. Add the stock, the eggplant, lime juice and the parsley. Mix and cook over medium heat for 30 minutes. Divide into bowls and serve.
Enjoy!

Nutrition: calories 300, fat 4, fiber 7, carbs 8, protein 9

Beans and Cauliflower Stew

Preparation time: 10 minutes
Cooking time: 1 hour
Servings: 4

Ingredients:

- 1 cup black beans, soaked for 12 hours and drained
- 4 garlic cloves, minced
- 1 yellow onion, chopped
- ½ teaspoon garam masala
- 1-inch fresh grated ginger
- ½ teaspoon ground coriander
- ½ teaspoon cayenne pepper
- 1 teaspoon ground turmeric
- 2 cups unsweetened coconut shredded
- 2 tomatoes, pureed
- 1 ½ cups cauliflower florets
- 2 cups veggie stock
- A pinch of salt and black pepper
- 1 teaspoon olive oil
- ½ teaspoon cumin seeds

Directions:

Heat up a pot with the oil over medium heat. Add cumin, onion, ginger and garlic, stir and cook for 5 minutes. Add the beans, coriander, cayenne pepper, turmeric, coconut, tomatoes, cauliflower, salt, pepper and stock. Stir, cover the pot, cook over medium heat for 1 hour, divide into bowls and serve.
Enjoy!

Nutrition: calories 219, fat 8, fiber 8, carbs 12, protein 8

Squash and Chickpea Stew

Preparation time: 10 minutes
Cooking time: 1 hour
Servings: 2
Ingredients:

- 2 cups chickpeas, soaked overnight and drained
- 2 cups veggie stock
- 1 butternut squash, cubed
- 1 teaspoon olive oil
- ½ cup red onion, chopped
- ½ teaspoon cumin seeds
- 4 garlic cloves minced
- 1 green chili, chopped
- ½ inch fresh grated ginger
- ½ teaspoon garam masala
- ¼ teaspoon ground turmeric
- 1 teaspoon lime juice
- 2 tomatoes chopped
- A pinch of salt and black pepper
- A pinch of cayenne pepper
- 1 cup spinach
- 1 tablespoon chopped cilantro

Directions:

Heat up a pot with the oil over medium heat. Add cumin, chili, garlic, ginger and onions, stir and sauté them for 5 minutes. Add turmeric, garam masala, lime juice, spinach, tomato, stir and cook for 5 minutes. Add chickpeas, stock, salt, pepper, cayenne, squash, stir, simmer over medium heat for 45 minutes. Add the spinach and the cilantro, mix and cook for 5 minutes more then divide into bowls and serve.
Enjoy!
Nutrition: calories 281, fat 6, fiber 4, carbs 8, protein 12

Black Beans and Cocoa Chili

Preparation time: 10 minutes
Cooking time: 1 hour and 15 minutes
Servings: 6
Ingredients:

- 1 red bell pepper, chopped
- 2 teaspoons olive oil
- 2 yellow onions, chopped
- 6 garlic cloves, minced
- 1 green bell pepper, chopped
- 24 ounces canned black beans, drained
- 6 cups veggie stock
- 1 tablespoon cocoa powder
- 2 tablespoons chili powder, mild
- 2 teaspoons ground cumin
- ½ teaspoon chipotle powder
- 2 teaspoons smoked paprika
- 30 ounces canned tomatoes, chopped
- 1/3 cup quinoa
- 1½ cups corn
- A pinch of salt and black pepper

Directions:

Heat up a pot with the oil over medium heat. Add onions, stir and cook them for 5 minutes. Add red peppers, green bell peppers, garlic, stock, beans, cocoa powder, chili powder, cumin, chipotle powder, paprika and tomatoes. Stir everything together, cover and cook over medium heat for about 50 minutes. Add quinoa, corn, salt and pepper, stir, cook for 10-15 minutes more then divide into bowls and serve.
Enjoy!
Nutrition: calories 300, fat 2, fiber 10, carbs 15, protein 11

Black Bean Soup

Preparation time: 10 minutes
Cooking time: 1 hour
Servings: 6

Ingredients:

- 1 yellow onion, chopped
- 1 pound black beans, soaked for a few hours and drained
- 2 teaspoons ground cumin
- 6 cups veggie stock
- 12 ounces corn
- ¼ teaspoon chipotle powder
- 1 cup salsa

Directions:
Pour the stock into a pot and heat over medium. Add the onion, the beans, cumin, corn, chipotle powder and salsa, mix, bring to a boil and cook for 1 hour. Ladle into bowls and serve.
Enjoy!

Nutrition: calories 224, fat 2, fiber 12, carbs 10, protein 17

Barley Soup

Preparation time: 10 minutes
Cooking time: 1 hour and 10 minutes
Servings: 4

Ingredients:

- 2 yellow onions, chopped
- ¼ cup pearl barley
- 4 cups veggie stock
- 6 ounces brown mushrooms, halved
- A pinch of salt and black pepper
- 3 garlic cloves, minced
- 2 teaspoons chopped thyme
- 12 ounces cabbage, shredded
- ½ teaspoon smoked paprika
- ½ teaspoon hot paprika
- 4 cups water
- 16 ounces canned black beans, drained and rinsed
- 1 tablespoon lemon juice

Directions:
In a pot, mix stock with the barley. Stir, bring to a simmer over medium heat and cook for 30 minutes. Add mushrooms, cabbage, smoked paprika, hot paprika, garlic, onions, salt, pepper, thyme, beans, lemon juice and water. Stir, cover the pot, cook over medium heat for 40 minutes more. Ladle into bowls and serve.
Enjoy!

Nutrition: calories 100, fat 0, fiber 7, carbs 19, protein 5

Sweet Potato Soup

Preparation time: 10 minutes
Cooking time: 35 minutes
Servings: 4

Ingredients:
- 2 tablespoons olive oil
- 4 garlic cloves, minced
- 1 yellow onion, chopped
- 2 tablespoons chopped cilantro
- 1 small red chili, chopped
- 2 teaspoons ground cumin
- A pinch of salt and black pepper
- 1 teaspoon sweet paprika
- 1 teaspoon coriander seeds
- 1 pound sweet potatoes, cubed
- 3 cups water
- Juice of ½ lime
- 10 ounces canned black beans, drained and rinsed
- 2 cups tomatoes, chopped
- A handful parsley, chopped

Directions:
Heat up a pot with the oil over medium heat then add the onion, stir and cook for 5 minutes. Add chili, garlic, salt, pepper, cilantro, cumin, coriander, paprika, sweet potatoes, tomatoes, black beans, water and lime juice. Stir, bring to a simmer and cook for 30 minutes. Add parsley, ladle into bowls and serve.
Enjoy!

Nutrition: calories 203, fat 5, fiber 4, carbs 7, protein 8

Beet Soup

Preparation time: 10 minutes
Cooking time: 45 minutes
Servings: 4

Ingredients:
- 2 tablespoons olive oil
- 1 yellow onion, chopped
- A pinch of salt and black pepper
- 1 carrot, grated
- 2 beets, grated
- 1 small green cabbage, shredded
- 4 garlic cloves, minced
- 3 tablespoons apple cider vinegar
- 10 porcini mushrooms, dried
- 1½ tablespoons tomato paste
- 5 cups water
- 1 tablespoons chopped parsley

Directions:
Heat up a pot with the oil over medium heat, add onion, stir and cook for 5 minutes. Add beets, carrot, garlic, cabbage, mushrooms, tomato paste, vinegar, salt, pepper and water. Stir, bring to a boil and cook over medium heat for 40 minutes. Add parsley, stir, ladle into bowls and serve.
Enjoy!

Nutrition: calories 300, fat 5, fiber 9, carbs 8, protein 7

Chicken and Zucchini Meatballs

Preparation time: 10 minutes
Cooking time: 10 minutes
Servings: 4

Ingredients:

- 1 cup shredded zucchini
- 2 pounds ground chicken
- 2 tablespoons harissa
- 1 garlic clove, minced
- ¼ cup chopped green onions
- 1 egg
- 2 tablespoons balsamic vinegar
- 1 tablespoon maple syrup
- A pinch of salt and black pepper

Directions:

In a bowl, mix chicken with zucchini, green onions, egg, garlic clove, harissa, balsamic vinegar, salt, pepper and maple syrup, stir well and shape into medium meatballs. Heat up a pan with the oil over medium heat, add the meatballs and cook them for 5 minutes on each side. Divide between plates and serve for lunch with a side salad.
Enjoy!

Nutrition: calories 200, fat 2, fiber 2, carbs 14, protein 12

Crispy Cod

Preparation time: 10 minutes
Cooking time: 15 minutes
Servings: 2

Ingredients:

- 1 egg white
- ½ cup red quinoa, already cooked
- 2 teaspoons whole wheat flour
- 4 teaspoons lemon juice
- ½ teaspoon smoked paprika
- 3 teaspoons olive oil
- 2 medium black cod fillets, skinless and boneless
- 1 red plum, pitted and chopped
- 2 teaspoons raw honey
- ¼ teaspoon black peppercorns, crushed
- 2 teaspoons parsley
- ¼ cup water

Directions:

In a bowl, whisk together 1 teaspoon lemon juice with egg white, flour and ¼ teaspoon paprika. Put quinoa in a bowl and mix it with 1/3 of egg white mix. Put the fish into the bowl with the remaining egg white mix, toss to coat, then dip the fish in quinoa mix and also toss to coat. Heat up a pan with 1 teaspoon oil over medium heat and add peppercorns, honey and plum. Stir, bring to a simmer and cook for 1 minute. Add the rest of the lemon juice, the rest of the paprika and the water to the pan, stir well and simmer for 5 minutes. Add parsley, stir, take the sauce off the heat and set aside for now. Heat up a pan with the rest of the olive oil over medium heat, add the coated fish cook for 3 minutes. Move the fish to a lined sheet tray and bake in the oven at 400 degrees F for 10 minutes more. Divide between plates, drizzle the plums sauce all over and serve.
Enjoy!

Nutrition: calories 324, fat 1, fiber 2, carbs 17, protein 22

Greek Sea Bass Mix

Preparation time: 10 minutes
Cooking time: 22 minutes
Servings: 2

Ingredients:

- 2 sea bass fillets, boneless
- 1 garlic clove, minced
- 5 cherry tomatoes, halved
- 1 tablespoon chopped parsley
- 2 shallots, chopped
- Juice of ½ lemon
- 1 tablespoon olive oil
- 8 ounces baby spinach
- Cooking spray

Directions:
Grease a baking dish with cooking oil then add the fish, tomatoes, parsley and garlic. Drizzle the lemon juice over the fish, cover the dish and place it in the oven at 350 degrees F. Bake for 15 minutes and then divide between plates. Heat up a pan with the olive oil over medium heat, add shallot, stir and cook for 1 minute. Add spinach, stir, cook for 5 minutes more, add to the plate with the fish and serve.
Enjoy!

Nutrition: calories 210, fat 3, fiber 6, carbs 10, protein 24

Creamy Asparagus Soup

Preparation time: 10 minutes
Cooking time: 0 minutes
Servings: 2

Ingredients:

- 8 ounces white mushrooms
- 12 asparagus spears, trimmed
- 1 avocado, pitted and peeled
- A pinch of salt and white pepper
- 1 yellow onion, peeled and chopped
- 3 cups water

Directions:
In your blender, add the mushrooms with asparagus, avocado, onion, water, salt and pepper. Pulse well, divide into soup bowls and serve right away. Heat if desired.
Enjoy!

Nutrition: calories 176, fat 3, fiber 9, carbs 16, protein 9

Mushroom Cream

Preparation time: 10 minutes
Cooking time: 0 minutes
Servings: 2

Ingredients:

- 2 tablespoons coconut aminos
- 1 tablespoon lime juice
- A pinch of sea salt and white pepper
- 1 cup white mushrooms
- 1 garlic clove, peeled
- 1 small yellow onion, chopped
- 2 cups cashew milk, unsweetened

Directions:

In your blender, mix mushrooms with garlic, onion, cashew milk, salt, pepper, lime juice and coconut aminos and pulse really well. Divide into soup bowls and serve right away.
Enjoy!

Nutrition: calories 191, fat 2, fiber 6, carbs 14, protein 7

Tomato Cream

Preparation time: 10 minutes
Cooking time: 0 minutes
Servings: 2

Ingredients:

- 3 sun-dried tomato sliced
- 2 celery stalks, chopped
- 3 big tomatoes, chopped
- ½ teaspoon powdered onion
- 2 basil springs, chopped
- ½ teaspoon garlic powder
- 1 small avocado, pitted and peeled
- A pinch of sea salt and white pepper

Directions:

In your blender, add the tomatoes with celery, onion powder, garlic powder, basil, avocado, salt and pepper and pulse really well. Add sun-dried tomatoes and blend again until smooth. Divide into soup bowls and serve.
Enjoy!

Nutrition: calories 167, fat 11, fiber 9, carbs 14, protein 4

Grape Gazpacho

Preparation time: 5 minutes
Cooking time: 0 minutes
Servings: 4

Ingredients:

- 1 cup white grapes, seedless and halved
- 1 teaspoon sesame oil
- 2 cups almond milk, unsweetened
- 1 small cucumber, chopped
- A pinch of salt and white pepper
- 1 tablespoon chives, chopped for garnish
- Ice cubes for serving

Directions:

In your blender, mix grapes with cucumber, almond milk, sesame oil, salt and pepper. Pulse really well. Divide into soup bowls, add ice cubes, sprinkle chopped chives all over and serve. Enjoy!

Nutrition: calories 152, fat 2, fiber 4, carbs 7, protein 6

Mushroom, Avocado and Tomato Cream

Preparation time: 3 hours and 10 minutes
Cooking time: 0 minutes
Servings: 3

Ingredients:

- 1 yellow onion
- 1 tablespoon agave nectar
- 1 tablespoon balsamic vinegar
- 4 tablespoons extra-virgin olive oil
- 1 teaspoon olive oil
- 12 ounces mushrooms, sliced
- 1 tomato, chopped
- 1 avocado, pitted, peeled and roughly chopped
- 1 garlic clove, minced
- A pinch of salt and black pepper
- 1½ cups water

Directions:

In a bowl, mix mushrooms with agave, vinegar, garlic, salt, pepper and 3 tablespoons olive oil. Toss well then transfer this to your dehydrator and dehydrate the mushrooms for 3 hours. Pour the mushrooms in your blender, add onion, 1 tablespoon oil, tomato, avocado, salt, pepper and the water. Pulse very well until smooth. Divide into soup bowls, drizzle 1 teaspoon oil on top and serve.
Enjoy!

Nutrition: calories 199, fat 4, fiber 6, carbs 14, protein 7

Veggie Tangine

Preparation time: 10 minutes
Cooking time: 35 minutes
Servings: 6

Ingredients:

- 2 tablespoons olive oil
- 1 yellow onion, chopped
- 1 parsnip, chopped
- 2 garlic cloves, minced
- 1 teaspoon cumin, ground
- ½ teaspoon fresh grated ginger
- ½ teaspoon ground cinnamon
- A pinch of salt and cayenne pepper
- 3 tablespoons tomato paste
- 2 sweet potatoes, peeled and cubed
- 2 purple potatoes, peeled and cubed
- 2 bunches baby carrots, peeled
- 1-quart veggie stock
- 2 tablespoons lemon juice
- 2 cups chopped kale
- ¼ cup chopped cilantro

Directions:

Place a pot with the oil over medium heat, add the onion, stir and sauté for 5 minutes. Add the parsnip, toss and cook for 3 minutes more. Add the garlic, ginger, cumin, salt, cayenne, cinnamon and tomato paste, toss and cook for 2 minutes. Add baby carrots, purple potatoes sweet potatoes and stock. Mix well and cover the pot, reduce heat to medium-low and cook for 20 minutes. Add lemon juice and kale, mix and cook for 1-2 minutes. Divide into bowls and serve with chopped cilantro on top.
Enjoy!

Nutrition: calories 212, fat 7, fiber 7, carbs 12, protein 7

Shrimp Stir-Fry

Preparation time: 10 minutes
Cooking time: 10 minutes
Servings: 4

Ingredients:

- ¼ cup coconut aminos
- 2 tablespoons raw honey
- 2 teaspoons sesame oil
- 2 tablespoons hemp seeds
- 2 tablespoons olive oil
- 1 pound shrimp, peeled and deveined
- 1 yellow onion, chopped
- 1 red bell pepper, sliced
- 1 yellow squash, peeled and cubed
- 4 ounces shiitake mushrooms, sliced
- 2 garlic cloves, minced
- 2 cups rainbow chard

Directions:

In a bowl, mix the aminos with the honey, sesame oil and hemp seeds. Heat up a pan with the olive oil over medium-high heat, add the onion, stir and cook for 2 minutes. Add the bell pepper, squash, mushrooms and garlic, stir and cook for 5 minutes. Add the shrimp and the coconut aminos then mix, cook for 4 minutes more, take off heat and add the chard. Mix well and divide everything into bowls and serve.
Enjoy!

Nutrition: calories 211, fat 6, fiber 4, carbs 11, protein 8

Black Rice Mix

Preparation time: 10 minutes
Cooking time: 10 minutes
Servings: 4

Ingredients:

- 2 carrots, chopped
- 2 tablespoons coconut oil
- 1 yellow onion, chopped
- 1 bunch scallions, sliced
- 2 garlic cloves, minced
- 1 cup sliced snap peas
- 1 tablespoon fresh grated ginger
- 3 cups black rice, cooked
- 2 teaspoons sesame oil
- 3 tablespoons coconut aminos
- 1 teaspoon sriracha
- 2 eggs, whisked
- 1 tablespoon hemp seeds

Directions:
Heat up a pan with the coconut oil over medium heat then add the onion, carrots and scallions. Stir and cook for 5 minutes. Add the garlic, snap peas and ginger. Stir and cook for 2 minutes more. Add the rice, aminos, the sriracha and sesame oil, stir and cook for 2 minutes. Add the eggs, mix and cook until they are done (about 1-2 minutes). Divide into bowls, sprinkle hemp seeds on top and serve.
Enjoy!

Nutrition: calories 182, fat 2, fiber 9, carbs 21, protein 11

Chard and Lentil Soup

Preparation time: 10 minutes
Cooking time: 30 minutes
Servings: 4

Ingredients:

- 1 yellow onion, chopped
- 2 tablespoons olive oil
- 2 carrots, chopped
- 2 garlic cloves, minced
- 1 teaspoon ground cumin
- ½ teaspoon ground ginger
- ½ teaspoon ground turmeric
- ½ teaspoon red chili flakes
- A pinch of salt and black pepper
- 15 ounces canned tomatoes, chopped
- 1 cup red lentils
- 2 quarts veggie stock
- 1 bunch chard, roughly chopped

Directions:
Heat up a pot with the oil over medium heat. Add the onion and carrot, stir and cook for 7 minutes. Add chili flakes, garlic, cumin, ginger, turmeric, salt and pepper, stir and cook for 1 more minute. Add tomatoes, stir and cook for another 5 minutes. Add the lentils and stock, stir, bring to a boil, reduce heat to medium-low and simmer for 10 minutes. Add the chard, toss, cook for 5 minutes, ladle into bowls and serve.
Enjoy!

Nutrition: calories 181, fat 4, fiber 4, carbs 9, protein 11

Salmon and Quinoa Salad

Preparation time: 10 minutes
Cooking time: 20 minutes
Servings: 4

Ingredients:

- 1 cup white quinoa, rinsed
- 1 bunch kale, torn
- 2 tablespoon lemon juice
- 1 carrot, sliced
- 2 cups water
- 2 garlic cloves, minced
- 1 tablespoon olive oil
- A pinch of salt and black pepper
- 2 cups canned chickpeas, drained and rinsed
- ¼ cup dried currants
- 1 tablespoons hemp seeds
- 4 salmon fillets, skin-on and boneless

For the sauce:
- ½ cup water
- ¼ cup tahini paste
- 1 tablespoon lemon juice
- ½ cup coconut cream

Directions:
Put the quinoa and 2 cups water in a pot then bring to a simmer over medium heat, cook for 15 minutes, set aside for another 10 minutes to cool and then fluff with a fork. In a salad bowl, mix the cooked quinoa with carrot, garlic, chickpeas, currants, kale, lemon juice and hemp seed and toss. In another bowl, combine½ cup water with tahini, 1 tablespoon lemon juice and coconut cream, whisk well and pour over the quinoa mix. Toss the mix and set aside. Heat up a pan with the olive oil over medium-high heat, add the salmon, season with salt and pepper and cook for 3-4 minutes on each side. Divide between plates, add the quinoa mix on the side and serve.
Nutrition: calories 211, fat 14, fiber 10, carbs 16, protein 12

Easy Shrimp Mix

Preparation time: 10 minutes
Cooking time: 15 minutes
Servings: 4

Ingredients:

- 1 pound shrimp, deveined and peeled
- 2 teaspoons olive oil
- 6 tablespoons lemon juice
- 3 tablespoons chopped dill
- 1 tablespoon chopped oregano
- 2 garlic cloves, chopped
- Salt and black pepper to the taste
- ¾ cup coconut cream
- ½ pounds cherry tomatoes
- 2 cucumbers, sliced
- 1 red onion, sliced
- 8 lettuce leaves

Directions:
In a bowl mix the shrimp with 2 tablespoons lemon juice, 1 tablespoon dill, 1 tablespoon oregano and 1 teaspoon oil and set aside for 10 minutes. In another bowl, mix ¼ cup coconut cream with 1 tablespoon dill, half of the garlic, 2 tablespoons lemon juice, cucumber, salt and pepper. In a third bowl, whisk together½ cup cream with the rest of the lemon juice, the rest of the garlic and the rest of the dill. In a bowl, mix tomatoes with onion and 1 teaspoon olive oil and toss. Heat up your kitchen grill over medium-high heat and grill tomatoes and shrimp for 5 minutes. Divide between plates, add cucumber salad, onions, tomatoes, shrimp and the lettuce leaves on top
Nutrition: calories 273, fat 6, fiber 6, carbs 10, protein 11

Salmon and Sweet Potato Mix

Preparation time: 10 minutes
Cooking time: 0 minutes
Servings: 4

Ingredients:

- 1½ pounds sweet potatoes, baked and cubed
- 1 tablespoon olive oil
- 4 ounces smoked salmon, chopped
- 1 tablespoon chopped chives
- 2 teaspoons horseradish
- ¼ cup coconut cream
- Salt and black pepper to the taste

Directions:
In a bowl, whisk together the coconut cream with salt, pepper, horseradish and chives. Add salmon and potatoes, toss to coat and serve right away.
Enjoy!

Nutrition: calories 233, fat 6, fiber 5, carbs 37, protein 9

Cod and Tarragon Sauce

Preparation time: 10 minutes
Cooking time: 15 minutes
Servings: 4

Ingredients:

- 4 medium cod fillets, skinless and boneless
- 2 tablespoons mustard
- 1 tablespoon chopped tarragon
- 1 tablespoon capers, drained
- 4 tablespoons olive oil+ 1 teaspoon
- Salt and black pepper to the taste
- 2 cups lettuce leaves, torn
- 1 small red onion, sliced
- 1 small cucumber, sliced
- 2 tablespoons lemon juice
- 2 tablespoons water

Directions:
In a bowl, mix mustard with 2 tablespoons olive oil, tarragon, capers and water, whisk well and set aside. Heat up a pan with 1 teaspoon oil over medium-high heat. Season fish with salt and pepper to the taste then add to pan and cook for 6 minutes on each side. In a separate bowl, mix cucumber with onion, lettuce, lemon juice, 2 tablespoons olive oil, salt and pepper to the taste. Arrange the cod between plates, drizzle the tarragon sauce all over and serve with the cucumber salad on the side.
Enjoy!

Nutrition: calories 261, fat 8, fiber 1, carbs 8, protein 14

Shrimp and Mango Mix

Preparation time: 10 minutes
Cooking time: 0 minutes
Servings: 5

Ingredients:
- 2 tablespoons Dijon mustard
- 3 tablespoons white wine vinegar
- 6 tablespoons avocado mayonnaise
- 4 cucumbers, peeled and cubed
- 1 mango, peeled and cubed
- 3 tablespoons chopped dill
- 1 pound shrimp, cooked, peeled and deveined
- A pinch of salt and black pepper

Directions:
In a salad bowl, mix the cucumbers with the mango, shrimp, dill, salt and pepper and toss. Add the mustard, vinegar and mayonnaise and mix well then serve.
Enjoy!

Nutrition: calories 174, fat 3, fiber 2, carbs 4

Orange Chicken Salad

Preparation time: 10 minutes
Cooking time: 30 minutes
Servings: 4

Ingredients:
- 1 whole chicken, cut into medium pieces
- 4 scallions, chopped
- 2 celery ribs, chopped
- 1 cup chopped mandarin orange
- ¼ cup avocado mayonnaise
- ½ cup coconut cream
- 1 cup chopped cashews, toasted
- A pinch of salt and black pepper

Directions:
Put chicken pieces in a pot and add water to cover. Add a pinch of salt then bring to a boil over medium heat and cook for 25 minutes. Transfer to a cutting board, discard bones, shred meat and put in a bowl. Add celery, orange pieces, cashews, scallion, salt, pepper, mayo and the coconut cream, toss to coat and serve.
Enjoy!

Nutrition: calories 210, fat 3, fiber 3, carbs 16, protein 18

Brown Rice and Chicken Mix

Preparation time: 10 minutes
Cooking time: 10 minutes
Servings: 4

Ingredients:
- 1½ cups brown rice, cooked
- 1½ tablespoons stevia
- 1 cup chicken stock
- 2 tablespoon coconut aminos
- 4 ounces chicken breast boneless, skinless and cut into small pieces
- 1 egg
- 2 egg whites
- 2 scallions, chopped

Directions:
Put stock in a pot, heat up over medium-low heat and add coconut aminos and stevia, stir, bring to a boil, add the chicken and toss. In a bowl, mix the egg with egg whites, whisk well then add over the chicken mix. Sprinkle the scallions on top and cook for 3 minutes without stirring. Divide the rice into 4 bowls, add the chicken mix on top and serve.
Enjoy!

Nutrition: calories 231, fat 11, fiber 7, carbs 8, protein 9

Greek Chicken Breasts

Preparation time: 10 minutes
Cooking time: 30 minutes
Servings: 6

Ingredients:
- 6 chicken breast halves, skinless and boneless
- 2 teaspoons olive oil
- ½ cup vegetable stock
- 1 tablespoon chopped basil
- 2 teaspoons chopped thyme
- ½ cup chopped yellow onion
- 3 garlic cloves, minced
- ½ cup kalamata olives, pitted and sliced
- ¼ cup chopped parsley
- 3 cups chopped tomatoes

Directions:
Heat up a pan with the oil over medium heat, add chicken and cook for 6 minutes on each side. Transfer cooked chicken to a plate. Heat up the same pan used for the chicken over medium heat, add garlic, stir and cook for 1 minute. Add onion, tomatoes and the stock then stir and bring to a simmer. Cook for 10 minutes. Add basil, thyme and the chicken, mix and cook for 12 minutes. Add parsley, olives, salt and pepper, toss, divide between plates and serve.
Enjoy!

Nutrition: calories 221, fat 2, fiber 4, carbs 7, protein 8

Easy Chicken and Potato Mix

Preparation time: 10 minutes
Cooking time: 50 minutes
Servings: 4

Ingredients:

- 1 tablespoon olive oil
- 4 teaspoons garlic, minced
- A pinch of salt and black pepper
- ¼ teaspoon dried thyme
- 12 small red potatoes, halved
- Cooking spray
- 2 pounds chicken breast, skinless, boneless and cubed
- 1 cup sliced red onion
- ¾ cup vegetable stock
- ½ cup pepperoncini peppers, chopped
- 2 cups chopped tomato
- ¼ cup kalamata olives, pitted and halved
- 2 tablespoons chopped basil
- 14 ounces canned artichokes, drained and chopped

Directions:

In a baking dish, mix potatoes with 2 teaspoons garlic, olive oil, thyme, salt and pepper. Bake in the oven at 400 degrees F for 30 minutes. Heat up a pot over medium-high heat, grease with cooking spray, add chicken, season with salt and black pepper and cook for 5 minutes on each side then transfer to a plate. Heat up the pot again over medium heat, add onion, stir and cook for 5 minutes. Add stock and return the chicken to the pot. Add olives, pepperoncini and roasted potatoes, stir and cook for 3 minutes. Add the rest of the garlic, artichokes, basil and the tomatoes, stir, cook for 3 minutes. Divide between plates and serve.
Enjoy!

Nutrition: calories 221, fat 2, fiber 3, carbs 8, protein 11

Paprika Chicken Mix

Preparation time: 10 minutes
Cooking time: 30 minutes
Servings: 4

Ingredients:

- 1/3 cup mustard
- Salt and black pepper to the taste
- 1 cup yellow onion, chopped
- 1 and ½ cups chicken stock
- 4 chicken breasts, skinless and boneless
- ¼ teaspoon sweet paprika

Directions:

In a bowl, whisk the paprika with mustard, salt and pepper. Spread the mix over the chicken and rub well. Heat up a pan with the oil over medium-high heat, add chicken breasts and cook for 2 minutes on each side then transfer to a plate. Heat up the pan once again over medium-high heat, add stock, stir and bring to a simmer. Add onions, salt, pepper and return the chicken to the pan as well. Stir the mix and bring to a simmer over medium heat for 20 minutes, turning meat halfway. Divide between plates, drizzle the sauce over it and serve.
Enjoy!

Nutrition: calories 223, fat 8, fiber 1, carbs 3, protein 15

Veggie Lunch Salad

Preparation time: 10 minutes
Cooking time: 0 minutes
Servings: 4

Ingredients:
- 2 carrots, peeled and grated
- 1 avocado, pitted, peeled and chopped
- ½ green cabbage head, shredded
- 10 strawberries, halved
- Salt and black pepper to the taste
- ¼ teaspoon matcha powder
- 1 teaspoon maple syrup
- 2 tablespoons white wine vinegar
- 1 tablespoon Dijon mustard
- ¼ cup lemon juice
- ¾ cup olive oil

Directions:
In a bowl, whisk together the lemon juice with oil, vinegar, matcha tea powder, maple syrup, mustard, salt and pepper. In a salad bowl, mix avocado with cabbage, strawberries and carrots. Add lemon juice, oil, vinegar, matcha powder, maple syrup, mustard, salt and pepper. Toss well and serve for lunch.
Enjoy!

Nutrition: calories 211, fat 4, fiber 2, carbs 8, protein 7

Grilled Eggplant Lunch Salad

Preparation time: 10 minutes
Cooking time: 20 minutes
Servings: 4

Ingredients:
- 1 tomato, diced
- 1 eggplant, pricked
- A pinch of salt and black pepper
- ¼ teaspoon ground turmeric
- 1½ teaspoons red wine vinegar
- ½ teaspoon chopped oregano
- 3 tablespoons olive oil
- 2 garlic cloves, minced
- 3 tablespoons chopped parsley
- 2 tablespoons chopped capers

Directions:
Heat up your grill over medium-high heat, add eggplant, cook for 15 minutes, turning from time to time, scoop flesh, roughly chop and put in a bowl. Add salt, pepper to the taste, tomatoes, turmeric, garlic, vinegar, oregano, parsley, oil and capers, toss and serve.
Enjoy!

Nutrition: calories 192, fat 7, fiber 6, carbs 12, protein 7

Eggplant and Avocado Lunch Mix

Preparation time: 10 minutes
Cooking time: 10 minutes
Servings: 4

Ingredients:

- 1 eggplant, sliced
- 1 red onion, sliced
- 2 teaspoons olive oil
- 1 avocado, pitted and chopped
- 1 teaspoon mustard
- 1 tablespoon red wine vinegar
- 1 tablespoon chopped oregano
- 1 teaspoon raw honey
- A pinch of salt and black pepper
- 1 tablespoon chopped parsley
- Zest of 1 lemon

Directions:
Brush the onion slices and eggplant slices with the olive oil, place them on the preheated kitchen grill, cook for 5 minutes on each side and let cool down. Cut the veggies into cubes, put in a salad bowl, add avocado and toss. In a bowl, mix vinegar with mustard, oregano, honey, olive oil, salt and pepper, whisk well and add to the salad. Toss together and sprinkle the lemon zest and the parsley on top and serve.
Enjoy!

Nutrition: calories 212, fat 7, fiber 7, carbs 12, protein 7

Eggplant and Egg Mix

Preparation time: 10 minutes
Cooking time: 30 minutes
Servings: 4

Ingredients:

- 1 big purple eggplant, cubed
- ¼ cup olive oil
- 12 eggs, hard-boiled, peeled and cubed
- Juice of 1 lemon
- A pinch of salt and white pepper
- 1/3 cup pine nuts
- ¼ cup mustard
- 1 cup chopped sun-dried tomatoes
- 1 cup halved walnuts

Directions:
Spread eggplant cubes on a lined baking sheet. In a bowl, whisk together half of the lemon juice with the oil, salt and pepper. Pour the mix over the eggplant cubes, toss to coat, introduce in the oven at 400 degrees F and bake for 30 minutes. In a food processor, mix the rest of the lemon juice, mustard, salt, pepper, walnuts, tomatoes and pine nuts and pulse well. Put the eggs in a bowl, add eggplant cubes, mustard mix, toss to coat well and serve.
Enjoy!

Nutrition: calories 213, fat 8, fiber 3, carbs 12, protein 7

Stuffed Eggplants

Preparation time: 10 minutes
Cooking time: 50 minutes
Servings: 6

Ingredients:

- 6 baby eggplants, halved
- 2 garlic cloves, minced
- 1 pound ground turkey
- 1 tablespoon chopped oregano
- 1 tablespoon lemon juice
- ¼ teaspoon sweet paprika
- ¼ teaspoon ground turmeric
- A pinch of salt and black pepper
- 2 tablespoons olive oil

Directions:

Heat up a pan with the oil over medium heat, add the ground turkey, stir and cook for 5-6 minutes. Add the oregano, lemon juice, paprika, turmeric, salt and pepper, stir, and cook for 5-6 minutes more. Take off the heat, cool the mix down and stuff the eggplants with this mix. Arrange the stuffed eggplants on a lined baking sheet, bake in the oven at 400 degrees F for 30 minutes then divide between plates and serve.
Enjoy!

Nutrition: calories 185, fat 10, fiber 3, carbs 10, protein 16

Veggie Soup

Preparation time: 10 minutes
Cooking time: 30 minutes
Servings: 4

Ingredients:

- 1 yellow onion, chopped
- 2 carrots, chopped
- 6 mushrooms, chopped
- 1 red chili pepper, chopped
- 2 celery sticks, chopped
- 1 tablespoon coconut oil
- A pinch of salt and black pepper
- 4 garlic cloves, minced
- 4 ounces kale, chopped
- 1 cup canned tomatoes, chopped
- 1 zucchini, chopped
- 1-quart veggie stock
- A handful parsley, chopped for serving

Directions:

Heat up a pot with the oil over medium-high heat, add the celery, carrots, onion, salt and black pepper. Stir and cook for 2 minutes. Add chili pepper, garlic, and mushrooms, stir and cook for 2 minutes. Add tomatoes, stock, kale and zucchinis, stir then bring to a simmer. Cook for 25 minutes, divide into bowls, sprinkle the parsley on top and serve.
Enjoy!

Nutrition: calories 180, fat 2, fiber 2, carbs 7, protein 5

Shrimp Soup

Preparation time: 10 minutes
Cooking time: 30 minutes
Servings: 4

Ingredients:

- 5 tablespoons curry paste
- 1 tablespoon coconut oil
- 1 big chicken breast, cut into thin strips
- 4 tablespoons coconut aminos
- 2 cups chicken stock
- Juice of 1 lime
- 1 ½ cups coconut milk
- 1 pound shrimp, peeled and deveined
- ½ cup coconut cream
- 1 broccoli head, florets separated
- 1 zucchini, chopped
- 1 carrot, chopped
- 1 tablespoon parsley, chopped

Directions:

Heat up a pot with the oil over medium heat, add curry paste, stir and cook for 1 minute. Add chicken, stock and lime juice. Stir and cook for 2 minutes. Add coconut cream, aminos and coconut milk, stir and cook for 10 minutes. Add broccoli florets, carrots, shrimp and zucchini, stir and cook for 4 minutes. Ladle into bowls, top with parsley and serve.
Enjoy!

Nutrition: calories 190, fat 3, fiber 2, carbs 6, protein 8

Coconut Zucchini Cream

Preparation time: 10 minutes
Cooking time: 25 minutes
Servings: 4

Ingredients:

- 1 onion, chopped
- 3 zucchinis, cut into medium chunks
- 2 tablespoons coconut milk
- 2 garlic cloves, minced
- 4 cups chicken stock
- 2 tablespoons olive oil
- A pinch of sea salt and black pepper

Directions:

Heat up a pot with the oil over medium heat. Add zucchinis, garlic and onion, stir and cook for 5 minutes. Add stock, salt and pepper then stir. Bring to a boil, cover pot and simmer soup for 20 minutes. Mix with the coconut milk, blend using an immersion blender, ladle into bowls and serve.
Enjoy!

Nutrition: calories 312, fat 9, fiber 2, carbs 34, protein 7

Kale Soup

Preparation time: 10 minutes
Cooking time: 25 minutes
Servings: 4

Ingredients:
- 1 yellow onion, chopped
- 1 teaspoon olive oil
- 3 sweet potatoes, chopped
- 4 cups chicken stock
- 1 pound kale, chopped
- A pinch of sea salt and black pepper

Directions:
Heat up a pot with the oil over medium heat, add onion, stir and cook for 5 minutes. Add stock and sweet potatoes, stir, bring to a simmer and cook for 15 minutes. Blend using an immersion blender, add kale, salt and pepper, cook everything for 4 minutes more, ladle into bowls and serve.
Enjoy!

Nutrition: calories 200, fat 2, fiber 2, carbs 6, protein 8

French Soup

Preparation time: 10 minutes
Cooking time: 3 hours
Servings: 4

Ingredients:
- 2 tablespoons olive oil
- 5 yellow onions, cut into halves and then sliced
- Black pepper to the taste
- 5 cups vegetable stock
- ¼ teaspoon ground turmeric
- A pinch of cayenne pepper
- 3 thyme springs, chopped
- 1 tablespoon tomato paste

Directions:
Heat up a pot with the oil over medium-high heat, add onions and thyme, stir and reduce heat to low. Cover and cook for 30 minutes. Uncover the pot and cook onions for 1 hour and 30 minutes more stirring often. Add tomato paste, cayenne, black pepper, turmeric and stock, stir, simmer soup for 1 hour more, ladle soup into bowls and serve.
Enjoy!

Nutrition: calories 200, fat 4, fiber 4, carbs 12, protein 8

Chicken and Pumpkin Stew

Preparation time: 10 minutes
Cooking time: 8 hours
Servings: 6

Ingredients:
- 2 carrots, chopped
- 5 garlic cloves, minced
- 2 celery sticks, chopped
- 2 onions, chopped
- 2 sweet potatoes, cubed
- 30 ounces canned pumpkin puree
- 2 quarts chicken stock
- 2 cups chicken meat, skinless, boneless and shredded
- A pinch of sea salt and black pepper
- ¼ teaspoon cayenne pepper
- ¼ cup ground arrowroot
- ½ pound baby spinach

Directions:
In your slow cooker, mix carrots with garlic, celery, onion, sweet potatoes, pumpkin puree, chicken, stock, salt, pepper, cayenne and ground arrowroot. Stir, cover and cook on Low for 8 hours. Uncover slow cooker, add spinach, stir, divide the stew into bowls and serve.
Enjoy!

Nutrition: calories 280, fat 3, fiber 3, carbs 6, protein 7

Eggplant and Tomato Stew

Preparation time: 10 minutes
Cooking time: 25 minutes
Servings: 3

Ingredients:
- 2 big tomatoes, chopped
- 1 eggplant, chopped
- 1 cup tomato paste
- 1 yellow onion, chopped
- A pinch of cayenne pepper
- 1 teaspoon ground cumin
- A pinch of salt and black pepper
- ½ cup vegetable stock

Directions:
Put the stock in a small pot and heat it up over medium heat. Add the tomato paste, cayenne, salt, pepper, tomatoes, eggplant and onion. Stir, bring to a simmer, cover the pot and cook stew for 25 minutes. Divide into bowls and serve.
Enjoy!

Nutrition: calories 210, fat 5, fiber 5, carbs 14, protein 8

Lemony Salmon Mix

Preparation time: 10 minutes
Cooking time: 1 hour
Servings: 2

Ingredients:
- 1 big salmon fillet, halved
- 2 teaspoons olive oil
- A pinch of salt and black pepper

For the relish:
- 1 tablespoon lemon juice
- 1 shallot, chopped
- 1 Meyer lemon, cut in wedges and then thinly sliced
- 2 tablespoons parsley, chopped
- ¼ cup olive oil

Directions:
Arrange the salmon on a lined baking dish, drizzle 2 teaspoons olive oil, season with sea salt and black pepper and rub the seasoning into the fish. Place in the oven at 370 degrees F and bake for 1 hour. In a bowl, mix shallot with the lemon juice, salt and black pepper, stir and leave aside for 10 minutes. In another bowl, whisk together the marinated shallot with lemon slices, some salt, pepper, parsley and ¼ cup oil. Cut salmon in chunks, divide between plates, top with lemon relish and serve.
Enjoy!

Nutrition: calories 200, fat 8, fiber 3, carbs 6, protein 10

Easy Cod Fillets

Preparation time: 10 minutes
Cooking time: 20 minutes
Servings: 4

Ingredients:
- 1 tablespoon chopped parsley
- 4 medium cod filets
- ¼ cup oil+ 2 tablespoons
- 2 garlic cloves, minced
- 2 tablespoons lemon juice
- 1 teaspoon Dijon mustard
- 1 shallot, chopped
- A pinch of salt and black pepper

Directions:
In a bowl, whisk together the mustard with ¼ cup oil, garlic, parsley, shallot, lemon juice, salt and pepper. Heat up a pan with the rest of the oil over medium-high heat. Add fish fillets, season them with salt and black pepper and cook for 4 minutes on each side. Spread mustard mix over the fish, transfer everything to a lined baking sheet and place in the oven at 425 degrees F. Bake for 10 minutes, divide between plates and serve with a side salad
Enjoy!

Nutrition: calories 210, fat 12, fiber 6, carbs 9, protein 12

Salmon and Salsa

Preparation time: 15 minutes
Cooking time: 10 minutes
Servings: 4

Ingredients:

- 4 medium salmon fillets, boneless
- 2 teaspoons olive oil
- 4 teaspoons lemon juice
- 1 garlic clove, minced
- 1 teaspoon sweet paprika
- A pinch of salt and black pepper

For the salsa:

- ¼ cup chopped green onions
- 1 cup chopped red bell pepper
- 4 teaspoons chopped oregano
- 1 small habanero pepper, chopped
- 1 garlic clove, minced
- ¼ cup lemon juice

Directions:

In a bowl, mix red bell pepper with habanero, green onion, ¼ cup lemon juice, 1 garlic clove, oregano, salt and black pepper. In a separate large bowl, mix paprika, olive oil, 1 garlic clove and 4 teaspoons lemon juice. Stir, add the fish, rub it with the seasoning mix and leave aside for 10 minutes. Put the fish on the preheated grill over medium-high heat, season with sea salt and black pepper then cook for 5 minutes on each side. Divide between plates, top with the salsa and serve.
Enjoy!

Nutrition: calories 210, fat 3, fiber 2, carbs 13, protein 8

Wrapped Salmon

Preparation time: 10 minutes
Cooking time: 20 minutes
Servings: 4

Ingredients:

- 6 cabbage leaves, sliced in half
- 4 medium salmon steaks, skinless
- 2 red bell peppers, chopped
- 2 tablespoons coconut oil
- 1 yellow onion, chopped
- A pinch of sea salt and black pepper

Directions:

Put some water in a pot, bring to a boil over medium-high heat, add cabbage leaves and blanch them for 2 minutes then transfer to a bowl filled with cold water to stop the cooking. Remove from the water and pat dry them then set aside. Season salmon steaks with salt and black pepper to the taste and wrap each in 3 cabbage leaf halves. Heat up a pan with the coconut oil over medium-high heat, add onion and bell pepper, stir and cook for 4 minutes. Add wrapped salmon and place pan in the oven at 350 degrees F. Bake for 12 minutes. Divide the wrapped salmon and veggies between plates and serve.
Enjoy!

Nutrition: calories 210, fat 8, fiber 5, carbs 22, protein 8

Side Dish Recipes

Balsamic Beets

Preparation time: 10 minutes
Cooking time: 1 hour
Servings: 4

Ingredients:
- 2 tablespoons balsamic vinegar
- 8 beets, cut into quarters
- 1 tablespoon olive oil
- A pinch of ground turmeric
- ¼ teaspoon cayenne pepper
- A pinch of salt and black pepper

Directions:
In a bowl, mix beets with vinegar, oil, turmeric, cayenne, salt and pepper. Toss well and spread on a lined baking sheet. Bake in the oven at 350 degrees F for 1 hour then divide between plates and serve as a side dish.
Enjoy!

Nutrition: calories 150, fat 3, fiber 3, carbs 10, protein 7

Kale Sauté

Preparation time: 10 minutes
Cooking time: 10 minutes
Servings: 4

Ingredients:
- 3 bunches kale, roughly chopped
- A drizzle of olive oil
- ½ cup veggie stock
- 1 tablespoon lemon juice
- 1 garlic clove, minced
- A pinch of cayenne pepper
- ¼ teaspoon smoked paprika
- Black pepper to the taste

Directions:
Heat up a pan with the oil over medium-high heat. Add the garlic and cook for 1 minute. Add the kale, stock, lemon juice, paprika, cayenne and black pepper. Mix and cook for 9 minutes more. Divide between plates and serve as a side dish.
Enjoy!

Nutrition: calories 150, fat 5, fiber 2, carbs 4, protein 3

Orange Turnips Mix

Preparation time: 10 minutes
Cooking time: 10 minutes
Servings: 4

Ingredients:

- 2 tablespoons orange juice
- Zest of 2 oranges
- 16 ounces turnips, thinly sliced
- 3 tablespoons olive oil
- 1 tablespoon chopped rosemary
- A pinch of salt and black pepper

Directions:

Heat up a pan with the oil over medium-high heat, add turnips, stir and cook for 4 minutes. Add orange juice, orange zest, salt, black pepper and rosemary. Stir, cook for 10 minutes more, divide between plates and serve as a side dish.
Enjoy!

Nutrition: calories 130, fat 9, fiber 2, carbs 12, protein 4

Fennel Side Salad

Preparation time: 10 minutes
Cooking time: 0 minutes
Servings: 4

Ingredients:

- 3 tablespoons lemon juice
- 1 pound fennel, chopped
- A pinch of sea salt and black pepper
- 1/8 teaspoon ground turmeric
- 2 tablespoons olive oil

Directions:

In a salad bowl, mix the fennel with the lemon juice, salt, pepper, turmeric and oil. Toss and serve as a side dish.
Enjoy!

Nutrition: calories 100, fat 7, fiber 4, carbs 9, protein 1

Squash and Apple Mix

Preparation time: 10 minutes
Cooking time: 30 minutes
Servings: 4

Ingredients:

- ½ teaspoon ground cinnamon
- 2 tablespoons olive oil
- 2 apples, peeled, cored and cubed
- 2 pounds butternut squash, peeled, seeded and cubed

Directions:
In a baking dish, mix apples with squash, cinnamon and oil and toss to coat. Place in the oven at 350 degrees F and roast for 30 minutes. Divide between plates and serve as a side dish.
Enjoy!

Nutrition: calories 170, fat 5, fiber 2, carbs 11, protein 7

Mushrooms and Turnips Mix

Preparation time: 10 minutes
Cooking time: 15 minutes
Servings: 4

Ingredients:

- 1 teaspoon fresh grated ginger
- 1 pound white mushrooms, sliced
- 1 bunch turnip greens, trimmed
- 2 garlic cloves, minced
- A pinch of salt and black pepper
- ½ cup raw almonds
- ¼ cup lime juice
- 2 tablespoons olive oil
- 1 tablespoon coconut aminos

Directions:
Heat up a pan with the oil over medium-high heat. Add mushrooms and turnip greens and stir then cook for 2 minutes. Add ginger, garlic, lime juice, almonds, coconut aminos, salt and black pepper. Stir, cook for 12 minutes more, divide between plates and serve.
Enjoy!

Nutrition: calories 120, fat 9, fiber 2, carbs 4, protein 5

Bell Pepper and Kale Mix

Preparation time: 10 minutes
Cooking time: 10 minutes
Servings: 4

Ingredients:
- 5 cups kale, torn
- A pinch of salt and black pepper
- 3 small red bell peppers, chopped
- 1 tablespoon chopped parsley
- 3 tablespoons water
- 1 tablespoon olive oil

Directions:
Heat up a pan with the oil over medium-high heat and add the bell pepper, kale, water, salt and pepper. Mix and cook for 10 minutes. Add the parsley, toss, divide between plates and serve. Enjoy!

Nutrition: calories 120, fat 6, fiber 10, carbs 7, protein 6

Kale and Chard Mix

Preparation time: 10 minutes
Cooking time: 15 minutes
Servings: 4

Ingredients:
- ½ pound brown mushrooms, sliced
- 5 cups roughly chopped kale
- 1 ½ tablespoons olive oil
- 3 cups chopped red chard
- 2 tablespoons vegetable stock
- A pinch of salt and black pepper

Directions:
Heat up a pan with the oil over medium heat, add mushrooms, stir and cook for 10 minutes. Add red chard, kale, stock, salt and pepper. Stir, cook for 10 minutes, divide between plates and serve. Enjoy!

Nutrition: calories 170, fat 6, fiber 6, carbs 9, protein 4

Chili Squash

Preparation time: 10 minutes
Cooking time: 40 minutes
Servings: 4

Ingredients:

- 2 pounds butternut squash, cut into medium cubes
- A drizzle of olive oil
- 1 teaspoon chili powder
- 1 teaspoon garlic powder
- 1 teaspoon sweet paprika
- Black pepper to the taste

Directions:
Spread squash cubes on a lined baking sheet then drizzle the oil, sprinkle with the chili powder, garlic powder, paprika and black pepper. Toss well and place in the oven to bake at 360 degrees F for 40 minutes. Divide between plates and serve as a side dish.
Enjoy!

Nutrition: calories 132, fat 2, fiber 2, carbs 4, protein 6

Bok Choy Mix

Preparation time: 10 minutes
Cooking time: 10 minutes
Servings: 4

Ingredients:

- 2 tablespoons olive oil
- 3 tablespoons coconut aminos
- 1-inch fresh ginger, grated
- A pinch of red pepper flakes
- 4 bok choy heads, cut into quarters
- 2 garlic cloves, minced
- 1 tablespoon sesame seeds, toasted

Directions:
Heat up a pan with the oil over medium heat then add coconut aminos, garlic, pepper flakes and ginger. Stir and cook for 4 minutes. Add the bok choy and sesame seeds, mix and cook for 6 minutes. Divide between plates and serve.
Enjoy!

Nutrition: calories 160, fat 2, fiber 2, carbs 4, protein 5

Pumpkin Mash

Preparation time: 10 minutes
Cooking time: 35 minutes
Servings: 4

Ingredients:

- 1 teaspoon ground cinnamon
- 1 cup unsweetened coconut, shredded
- 1 pumpkin, peeled, seeded and cubed
- ¼ cup coconut oil
- A pinch of sea salt and black pepper

Directions:
Put the pumpkin in a pot, add water to cover and heat up over medium-high heat. Cover and cook for 30 minutes then drain, add salt, pepper, coconut and oil. Stir and cook over medium heat for 3 minutes. Mash using a potato masher, add the cinnamon and mash well again. Divide between plates and serve as a side dish.
Enjoy!

Nutrition: calories 435, fat 24, fiber 4, carbs 21, protein 4

Baked Pumpkin Side Salad

Preparation time: 10 minutes
Cooking time: 30 minutes
Servings: 6

Ingredients:

- 1 tablespoon raw honey + 2 teaspoons
- 2 tablespoons olive oil + 2 teaspoons
- 21-ounces pumpkin, peeled, seeded and cubed
- 2 teaspoons sesame seeds
- 1 tablespoon lemon juice
- 2 teaspoons mustard
- 4 ounces baby spinach
- 2 tablespoons pine nuts, toasted
- A pinch of salt and black pepper
- Black pepper to the taste

Directions:
In a bowl, mix pumpkin with salt, black pepper, 2 teaspoons oil and 2 teaspoons honey. Mix to coat well and spread on a lined baking sheet then bake in the oven at 400 degrees F for 25 minutes. Sprinkle the sesame seeds all over the pumpkin and bake for 5 minutes more. Cool the pieces down and put them in a bowl. Add spinach to the bowl and toss. In another small bowl, whisk the lemon juice with 1 tablespoon honey, 2 tablespoon oil and mustard. Add the dressing to the salad, toss and serve as a side dish.
Enjoy!

Nutrition: calories 220, fat 8, fiber 2, carbs 24, protein 6

Rice and Peas

Preparation time: 10 minutes
Cooking time: 20 minutes
Servings: 4

Ingredients:

- 1 yellow bell pepper, chopped
- 1 tablespoon olive oil
- 1 yellow onion, chopped
- 1 carrot, grated
- 2 cups black rice
- 3 cups water
- ½ cup peas
- A pinch of salt and black pepper

Directions:
Heat up a pot with the oil over medium heat, add onion, stir and cook for 5 minutes. Add carrots, bell pepper, peas, rice, salt, pepper and water, stir, bring to a simmer and cook for 15 minutes. Divide between plates and serve as a side dish.
Enjoy!

Nutrition: calories 202, fat 3, fiber 3, carbs 11, protein 6

Simple Black Beans Mash

Preparation time: 10 minutes
Cooking time: 1 hour and 10 minutes
Servings: 4

Ingredients:

- 1½ cups yellow onion, chopped
- 2 pounds black beans, soaked for 12 hours and drained
- 4 garlic cloves, chopped
- 2 teaspoons oregano, dried
- 1 jalapeno, chopped
- A pinch of salt and black pepper
- 3 tablespoons olive oil
- 6 cups veggie stock

Directions:
Heat up a pot with the oil over medium-high heat then add the onion, stir and sauté for 5 minutes. Add the garlic, the beans, oregano, jalapeno, salt, pepper and stock. Stir and bring to a simmer, reduce heat to medium-low, cook for 1 hour. Blend using an immersion blender, divide between plates and serve as a side dish.
Enjoy!

Nutrition: calories 221, fat 5, fiber 8, carbs 10, protein 8

Orange Brussels Sprouts

Preparation time: 10 minutes
Cooking time: 15 minutes
Servings: 6

Ingredients:

- 2 pounds Brussels sprouts, trimmed and halved
- 1 tablespoon olive oil
- 1 teaspoon orange zest, grated
- ¼ cup orange juice
- A pinch of salt and black pepper

Directions:
Heat up a pot with the oil over medium-high heat, add the sprouts, stir and cook for 2-3 minutes. Add orange zest, orange juice, salt and pepper, stir and cook for 12 minutes. Divide between plates and serve as a side dish.
Enjoy!

Nutrition: calories 193, fat 6, fiber 8, carbs 26, protein 6

Balsamic Green Cabbage

Preparation time: 10 minutes
Cooking time: 15 minutes
Servings: 4

Ingredients:

- 1 cabbage head, shredded
- 1 yellow onion, chopped
- 2 teaspoons balsamic vinegar
- 3 garlic cloves, minced
- 1 tablespoon olive oil
- A pinch of salt and black pepper
- 2 teaspoons mustard

Directions:
Heat up a pan with the oil over medium heat then add the onion and garlic, stir and sauté for 5 minutes. Add the cabbage, vinegar, mustard, salt and pepper, stir and cook for 10 minutes. Divide between plates and serve as a side dish.
Enjoy!

Nutrition: calories 180, fat 6, fiber 3, carbs 12, protein 6

Chili Cauliflower Rice

Preparation time: 10 minutes
Cooking time: 20 minutes
Servings: 6

Ingredients:

- 1 cup chopped yellow onion
- 3 tablespoons olive oil
- 2 cups riced cauliflower
- ¾ cup crushed tomatoes
- 2 garlic cloves, minced
- 2 cups veggie stock
- ¼ cup chopped cilantro
- ½ teaspoon chili powder

Directions:
Heat up a pan with the oil over medium-high heat and add the onions and garlic. Stir and cook for 4 minutes. Add cauliflower rice, stock, salt, pepper tomatoes and chili powder then stir, cook for 15 minutes and take off the heat. Add the cilantro and mix briefly then divide between plates and serve.
Enjoy!

Nutrition: calories 200, fat 4, fiber 3, carbs 6, protein 8

Herbed Quinoa

Preparation time: 10 minutes
Cooking time: 15 minutes
Servings: 4

Ingredients:

- 2 cups quinoa
- 3 cups water
- Juice of 1 lemon
- A pinch of salt and black pepper
- A handful mixed parsley, cilantro and basil, chopped

Directions:
In a pot, mix the quinoa with water, lemon, salt and pepper. Bring to a boil and simmer over medium heat for 15 minutes. Take off the heat, add mixed herbs, stir and set aside for 10 minutes. Once cooled slightly, fluff with a fork, divide between plates and serve as a side dish.
Enjoy!

Nutrition: calories 202, fat 1, fiber 6, carbs 12, protein 10

Black Beans and Veggie Mix

Preparation time: 10 minutes
Cooking time: 1 hour and 5 minutes
Servings: 6

Ingredients:

- 1 teaspoon olive oil
- 16 ounces black beans, soaked and drained
- 12 ounces green bell pepper, chopped
- 12 ounces sweet onion, chopped
- 4 garlic cloves, minced
- 2 ½ teaspoons ground cumin
- 2 tablespoons tomato paste
- 2 quarts water
- A pinch of salt and black pepper

Directions:
Heat up a pot with the oil over medium-high heat and add the onion, bell pepper and garlic. Stir and cook for 5 minutes. Add the beans, cumin, tomato paste, salt, pepper and the water. Toss, bring to a simmer, reduce heat to medium and cook the beans mix for 1 hour. Divide between plates and serve as a side dish.
Enjoy!

Nutrition: calories 221, fat 5, fiber 4, carbs 9, protein 11

Green Beans and Mushroom Sauté

Preparation time: 10 minutes
Cooking time: 25 minutes
Servings: 6

Ingredients:

- 1 pound green beans, trimmed
- 8 ounces white mushrooms, sliced
- 1 yellow onion, chopped
- 2 tablespoons olive oil
- ½ cup veggie stock
- A pinch of salt and black pepper

Directions:
Heat up a big pan with the oil over medium-high heat and add the onion, stir and cook for 4 minutes. Add the stock and the mushrooms then stir and cook for 6 minutes more. Add green beans, salt and pepper. Toss and cook over medium heat for 15 minutes then divide everything between plates and serve as a side dish.
Enjoy!

Nutrition: calories 182, fat 4, fiber 5, carbs 6, protein 8

Mediterranean Rice

Preparation time: 10 minutes
Cooking time: 30 minutes
Servings: 4

Ingredients:
- ¼ cup olive oil
- 1 cup black rice
- 2 green onions, chopped
- 1½ cups chicken stock
- ½ sweet onion, chopped
- ½ cup chopped carrots
- 2 tablespoons coconut aminos
- 1 teaspoon garlic powder

Directions:
In a pot, mix the stock with the rice, stir, bring to a simmer over medium heat and cook for 20 minutes stirring often. Remove the rice from the pan and set aside. Heat up a pan with the oil over medium heat, add the green onions, the carrots, sweet onion, rice, garlic powder and coconut aminos and stir then cook for 10 minutes. Divide between plates and serve as a side dish. Enjoy!

Nutrition: calories 261, fat 6, fiber 15, carbs 10, protein 6

Cauliflower Mash

Preparation time: 10 minutes
Cooking time: 15 minutes
Servings: 4

Ingredients:
- 1½ cups veggie stock
- 1 cauliflower head, florets separated
- 2 teaspoons olive oil
- A pinch of salt and black pepper
- ½ teaspoon ground turmeric
- 3 chives, chopped

Directions:
Put the stock and the cauliflower in a pot and bring to a boil over medium heat. Cook for 15 minutes, drain, and transfer to a bowl then mash using a potato masher. Add the oil, salt, pepper, chives and turmeric. Stir really well, divide between plates and serve as a side dish. Enjoy!

Nutrition: calories 200, fat 4, fiber 6, carbs 7, protein 10

Creamy Rice

Preparation time: 10 minutes
Cooking time: 20 minutes
Servings: 4

Ingredients:
- 14 ounces coconut milk
- 1½ cups jasmine rice
- 1 tablespoon coconut cream
- ½ cup water
- A pinch of salt and white pepper

Directions:
In a pot, mix the rice with the coconut milk, coconut cream, water, salt and white pepper. Stir and bring to a simmer over medium heat for 20 minutes, stir one more time then divide between plates and serve as a side dish.
Enjoy!

Nutrition: calories 191, fat 5, fiber 4, carbs 11, protein 9

Mushroom and Cauliflower Rice

Preparation time: 10 minutes
Cooking time: 15 minutes
Servings: 6

Ingredients:
- 1½ cups cauliflower rice
- 2 tablespoons olive oil
- 4 ounces wild mushrooms, roughly chopped
- 3 shallots, chopped
- 8 ounces cremini mushrooms, roughly chopped
- 2 cups veggie stock
- A pinch of salt and black pepper
- 2 tablespoons chopped cilantro

Directions:
Heat up a pot with the oil over medium heat and add the cauliflower rice and shallots. Stir and cook for 5 minutes. Add stock, cremini mushrooms and wild mushrooms then stir and cook for 10 minutes more. Add the parsley, salt and pepper and mix. Divide between plates and serve.
Enjoy!

Nutrition: calories 189, fat 3, fiber 4, carbs 9, protein 8

Simple Broccoli Stir-Fry

Preparation time: 10 minutes
Cooking time: 12 minutes
Servings: 4

Ingredients:

- 6 garlic cloves, minced
- 1 broccoli head, florets separated
- ½ cup veggie stock
- 1 tablespoon olive oil
- 1 tablespoon balsamic vinegar
- A pinch of salt and black pepper

Directions:

Heat up a pan with the oil over medium heat, add the garlic, stir and cook for 5 minutes. Add the broccoli, stock, vinegar, salt and pepper. Mix and cook for 7-8 minutes more then divide between plates and serve as a side dish.
Enjoy!

Nutrition: calories 182, fat 6, fiber 3, carbs 8, protein 6

Glazed Baby Carrots

Preparation time: 10 minutes
Cooking time: 15 minutes
Servings: 4

Ingredients:

- 1 tablespoon olive oil
- 3 pounds baby carrots, peeled
- 1 tablespoon maple syrup
- 1 teaspoon thyme, dried
- 1 tablespoon mustard
- 2 tablespoons veggie stock

Directions:

Heat up a pan with the oil over medium heat, add the baby carrots and brown them for 5-6 minutes. Add the maple syrup, thyme, stock and mustard, mix and cook for 10 minutes more. Divide between plates and serve.
Enjoy!

Nutrition: calories 180, fat 6, fiber 7, carbs 15, protein 6

Baked Asparagus

Preparation time: 10 minutes
Cooking time: 15 minutes
Servings: 4

Ingredients:

- 5 tablespoons olive oil
- 4 garlic cloves, minced
- 2 tablespoons chopped shallot
- Black pepper to the taste
- 1½ teaspoons balsamic vinegar
- 1½ pound asparagus, trimmed

Directions:
Spread the asparagus on a lined baking sheet, and drizzle the oil. Add the garlic, shallot, vinegar and black pepper then toss well and place in the oven. Bake at 450 degrees F for 15 minutes. Divide between plates and serve as a side dish.
Enjoy!

Nutrition: calories 132, fat 1, fiber 2, carbs 4, protein 4

Cucumber Salad

Preparation time: 1 hour
Cooking time: 0 minutes
Servings: 12

Ingredients:

- 2 cucumbers, chopped
- 2 tomatoes, chopped
- 1 tablespoon olive oil
- 1 yellow onion, chopped
- 1 jalapeno pepper, chopped
- 1 garlic clove, minced
- 1 teaspoon chopped parsley
- 2 tablespoons lime juice
- 2 teaspoons chopped cilantro
- ½ teaspoon dill, dried

Directions:
In a large salad bowl, mix the cucumbers with the tomatoes, onion, jalapeno, garlic, parsley, lime juice, cilantro, dill and oil. Mix well and keep in the fridge for 1 hour before serving as a side salad.
Enjoy!

Nutrition: calories 132, fat 3, fiber 1, carbs 7, protein 4

Eggplant Side Salad

Preparation time: 10 minutes
Cooking time: 10 minutes
Servings: 6

Ingredients:
- 1/3 cup homemade mayonnaise
- 2 tablespoons balsamic vinegar
- A pinch of salt and black pepper
- 1 tablespoon lime juice
- 2 big eggplants, sliced
- ¼ cup chopped parsley
- ¼ cup avocado oil

Directions:
In a small bowl, mix mayonnaise with vinegar, lime juice and black pepper. Stir well and set aside. Brush each eggplant slice with the avocado oil and season with salt and pepper. Place on the preheated grill over medium-high heat, and cook for 5 minutes on each side. Divide between plates. Drizzle the mayo mix all over, sprinkle parsley and serve as a side dish.
Enjoy!

Nutrition: calories 180, fat 2, fiber 2, carbs 8, protein 6

Barley Mix

Preparation time: 10 minutes
Cooking time: 45 minutes
Servings: 4

Ingredients:
- 1 tablespoon olive oil
- 1 yellow onion, chopped
- 4 parsnips, roughly chopped
- 1 tablespoon chopped sage
- 1 garlic clove, minced
- 14 ounces barley
- 6 cups hot veggie stock
- Salt and black pepper

Directions:
Heat up a pan with the oil over medium-high heat and add onion. Stir and cook for 5 minutes. Add parsnips, sage, garlic, barley and stock, stir well, bring to a simmer and cook for 40 minutes, divide between plates and serve.
Enjoy!

Nutrition: calories 286, fat 4, fiber 9, carbs 29, protein 4

Lentil and Chickpea Salad

Preparation time: 15 minutes
Cooking time: 30 minutes
Servings: 4

Ingredients:

- 7 ounces lentils, rinsed
- 3 tablespoons chopped capers
- Juice of 1 lemon
- Zest of 1 lemon
- 1 red onion, chopped
- 3 tablespoons olive oil
- 16 ounces canned chickpeas, drained
- 1 tablespoon chopped parsley
- A pinch of salt and black pepper

Directions:
Put lentils in a pot, add water to cover and bring to a simmer over medium heat. Boil for 30 minutes, drain and transfer to a bowl. Add capers, lemon juice, lemon zest, onion, oil, chickpeas, parsley, salt and pepper, toss and serve as a side dish.
Enjoy!

Nutrition: calories 212, fat 4, fiber 4, carbs 12, protein 6

Rice and Beans

Preparation time: 10 minutes
Cooking time: 1 hour
Servings: 6

Ingredients:

- 1 tablespoon olive oil
- 1 yellow onion, chopped
- 2 celery stalks, chopped
- 2 garlic cloves, minced
- 2 cups brown rice
- 1½ cup canned black beans, rinsed and drained
- 4 cups veggie stock
- Salt and black pepper to the taste

Directions:
Heat up a pan with the olive oil over medium heat, add celery and onion. Stir and cook for 8 minutes. Add beans and garlic, stir again and sauté them as well for about 5 minutes. Add rice, stock, salt and pepper. Stir, cover, cook for 45 minutes then divide between plates and serve. Enjoy!

Nutrition: calories 212, fat 3, fiber 2, carbs 2, protein 1

Green Onion and Tomato Mix

Preparation time: 10 minutes
Cooking time: 15 minutes
Servings: 6

Ingredients:

- 2 tablespoons olive oil
- 2 small bunches green onions, roughly chopped
- 2 tomatoes, chopped
- ½ cup chopped cilantro
- 5 drops hot sauce
- ½ cup lemon juice
- Salt and black pepper to the taste

Directions:
Heat up a pan with the oil over medium-high heat and add the tomatoes, hot sauce, salt and pepper. Mix well and cook for 5 minutes. Add the green onions, lemon juice and cilantro, toss and cook for 10 minutes over medium heat. Divide between plates and serve.
Enjoy!

Nutrition: calories 163, fat 6, fiber 2, carbs 7, protein 9

Quinoa and Greens Salad

Preparation time: 10 minutes
Cooking time: 0 minutes
Servings: 4

Ingredients:

- 1 cup quinoa, cooked
- 1 avocado, chopped
- 1 medium bunch collard greens, chopped
- 4 tablespoons walnuts, chopped
- 2 tablespoons white wine vinegar
- 1 tablespoon olive oil
- 1 tablespoon maple syrup

Directions:
In a bowl, mix the quinoa with the avocado, greens, walnuts, vinegar, oil and maple syrup, toss and serve as a side dish.
Enjoy!

Nutrition: calories 175, fat 3, fiber 3, carbs 5, protein 6

Avocado and Mango Side Salad

Preparation time: 10 minutes
Cooking time: 0 minutes
Servings: 4

Ingredients:

- 10 tablespoons roasted pepitas
- 1 handful cilantro, chopped
- 4 tablespoons chopped parsley
- 1 cup radish sprouts
- 2 avocados, peeled, pitted and chopped
- 2 mangos, peeled and chopped
- 3 tablespoons olive oil
- 4 tablespoons coconut cream
- 2 tablespoons lemon juice
- Salt and black pepper to the taste

Directions:

In a salad bowl, toss together the pepitas with the cilantro, parsley, radish sprouts, avocados, mangos, oil, cream, lemon juice, salt and pepper. Serve as a side dish.
Enjoy!

Nutrition: calories 200, fat 5, fiber 7, carbs 12, protein 3

Cabbage and Apple Side Salad

Preparation time: 1 hour and 10 minutes
Cooking time: 0 minutes
Servings: 4

Ingredients:

- 1 cup shredded cabbage
- 1 apple, cored and chopped
- 1 celery rib, chopped
- 1 carrot, grated
- 4 dates, chopped
- ¼ cup chopped cashews

For the salad dressing:

- 1 tablespoon lemon juice
- 2 garlic cloves, minced
- ¼ cup tahini paste
- 1 tablespoon apple cider vinegar
- 1 tablespoon agave nectar
- 2 tablespoons water
- 3 tablespoons olive oil
- 1 tablespoon chopped parsley
- A pinch of sea salt

Directions:

In a blender, mix lemon juice with the garlic, tahini paste, vinegar, agave nectar, water, olive oil, parsley and a pinch of salt and blend well. In a large salad bowl, mix the cabbage with celery, apple, carrots, dates and cashews. Add the salad dressing and toss then serve as a side dish.
Enjoy!

Nutrition: calories 140, fat 3, fiber 4, carbs 5, protein 14

Cucumber and Corn Salad

Preparation time: 10 minutes
Cooking time: 0 minutes
Servings: 4

Ingredients:

- 1 big cucumber, cut into chunks
- 1 cup corn
- 1 cup cherry tomatoes, halved
- 1 small red onion, chopped
- 3 tablespoons olive oil
- 4 teaspoons orange juice
- 1 teaspoon agave nectar
- Salt and black pepper to the taste
- ½ teaspoon ground cumin
- 1 tablespoon lemon juice

Directions:
In a bowl, mix the cucumber, corn, onion and tomatoes. In another bowl, whisk the orange juice with the oil, agave nectar, lemon juice, salt, pepper to the taste and cumin. Pour the dressing over the salad, toss to coat and serve.
Enjoy!

Nutrition: calories 110, fat 6, fiber 3, carbs 11, protein 8

Celery and Parsley Side Salad

Preparation time: 10 minutes
Cooking time: 0 minutes
Servings: 2

Ingredients:

- 1 tablespoon olive oil
- 1 teaspoon mustard
- 1 tablespoon lemon juice
- 2 cups roughly grated celery root
- Salt and black pepper to the taste
- 1 cup roughly chopped parsley

Directions:
In a bowl, mix the celery root with the mustard, oil, lemon juice, salt, pepper and parsley. Serve as a side salad.
Enjoy!

Nutrition: calories 138, fat 8, fiber 4, carbs 14, protein 3

Endive Salad

Preparation time: 10 minutes
Cooking time: 0 minutes
Servings: 4

Ingredients:

- 1 teaspoon minced shallot
- ¼ cup apple cider vinegar
- 1 teaspoon Dijon mustard
- 1 teaspoon agave nectar
- 3 endives, cut into medium pieces
- ¾ cup olive oil
- ½ apple, cored and roughly chopped
- 1 cup torn escarole leaves

Directions:

In a bowl, mix escarole leaves with endives, apple, shallot, vinegar, mustard, agave nectar and oil. Toss everything together well and serve.
Enjoy!

Nutrition: calories 120, fat 1, fiber 4, carbs 7, protein 7

Lettuce Side Salad

Preparation time: 10 minutes
Cooking time: 0 minutes
Servings: 4

Ingredients:

- ½ cup olive oil
- A pinch of salt and black pepper
- 2 tablespoons chopped shallot
- ¼ cup mustard
- Juice of 2 lemons
- ½ cup chopped basil
- Baby romaine lettuce heads, chopped
- 3 radicchio, sliced
- 3 endives, cut into medium pieces

Directions:

In a salad bowl, mix romaine lettuce with the radicchio and endives and stir gently. In another bowl, whisk the oil with salt, pepper, shallot, mustard, lemon juice and basil. Drizzle this over your salad, toss to coat and serve as a side salad.
Enjoy!

Nutrition: calories 190, fat 2, fiber 6, carbs 11, protein 7

Radish Salad

Preparation time: 10 minutes
Cooking time: 0 minutes
Servings: 4

Ingredients:

- 12 ounces tomatoes, chopped
- 1 cucumber, chopped
- 3 red onions, chopped
- 8 ounces red radishes, cut into wedges
- 3 tablespoons olive oil
- 1 teaspoon mustard
- 1 teaspoon mustard seeds
- Juice of 2 limes
- 2 teaspoons agave nectar
- 3 tablespoons chopped mint
- 1 red chili pepper, chopped

Directions:

In a salad bowl, mix tomatoes with cucumber, onions and radishes. In another bowl, whisk the mustard with mustard seeds, lime juice, agave nectar, chili pepper and mint. Pour the dressing over the salad, toss and serve as a side salad.
Enjoy!

Nutrition: calories 129, fat 3, fiber 2, carbs 8, protein 6

Cucumber and Radish Salad

Preparation time: 10 minutes
Cooking time: 0 minutes
Servings: 4

Ingredients:

- 1 cup sliced red onion
- 2 cups sliced radishes
- 1 garlic clove, minced
- A pinch of salt and black pepper
- 2 tablespoons balsamic vinegar
- 1 cup sliced cucumber
- 1 teaspoon chopped dill
- ½ cup olive oil

Directions:

In a salad bowl, mix onion with cucumber, radishes, garlic, salt, black pepper, oil, vinegar and dill. Toss to coat and serve.
Enjoy!

Nutrition: calories 110, fat 4, fiber 2, carbs 7, protein 7

Okra Side Salad

Preparation time: 40 minutes
Cooking time: 0 minutes
Servings: 4

Ingredients:

- 1 pound okra, cut into medium pieces
- A pinch of sea salt and black pepper
- 15 ounces canned black beans, drained
- 1 pound cherry tomatoes, halved
- 1 white onion, chopped
- 3 tablespoons olive oil
- 1 avocado, pitted, peeled and chopped

Directions:

Put okra in a salad bowl, add beans, onion, tomatoes, avocado, salt, black pepper and olive oil. Toss to coat and keep in the fridge for 30 minutes before serving as a side salad.
Enjoy!

Nutrition: calories 120, fat 1, fiber 1, carbs 8, protein 7

Tomato and Okra Side Salad

Preparation time: 10 minutes
Cooking time: 0 minutes
Servings: 4

Ingredients:

- 3 cups chopped okra
- 1 big tomato, chopped
- 3 celery stalks, chopped
- 1 onion, chopped
- 3 cups chopped cauliflower florets
- 1 yellow bell pepper, chopped
- A pinch of sea salt and black pepper
- Juice of 1 lemon
- ½ teaspoon red pepper flakes
- 1 teaspoon garlic powder

Directions:

In a salad bowl, mix okra with tomato, celery stalks, onion, cauliflower and bell pepper. Add the salt, black pepper, lemon juice, pepper flakes and garlic powder. Toss everything together and serve as a side dish.
Enjoy!

Nutrition: calories 80, fat 3, fiber 1, carbs 8, protein 5

Corn Side Salad

Preparation time: 10 minutes
Cooking time: 0 minutes
Servings: 4

Ingredients:

- 1 red bell pepper, thinly sliced
- 2 cups corn
- Juice of 1 lemon
- Zest of 1 lemon, grated
- 4 cups arugula
- A pinch of sea salt and black pepper

Directions:
In a salad bowl, mix arugula with the corn and bell pepper. Add the salt, pepper, lemon zest and lemon juice. Toss to coat evenly and serve as a side dish.
Enjoy!

Nutrition: calories 90, fat 2, fiber 1, carbs 7, protein 5

Bulgur Salad

Preparation time: 30 minutes
Cooking time: 0 minutes
Servings: 4

Ingredients:

- 1 cup bulgur
- 2 cups hot water
- A pinch of sea salt and black pepper
- 2 cups corn
- 1 cucumber, chopped
- 2 tablespoons lemon juice
- 2 tablespoons balsamic vinegar
- ¼ cup olive oil

Directions:
In a bowl, mix bulgur with the water, cover and set aside for 25 minutes. Uncover the bulgur and fluff with a fork. Transfer the bulgur to a salad bowl, add the corn and cucumber and toss. In a separate small bowl, whisk the oil with lemon juice, vinegar, salt and pepper. Add the dressing to your salad, toss to coat well and serve as a side dish.
Enjoy!

Nutrition: calories 253, fat 14, fiber 2, carbs 30, protein 4

Asparagus Salad

Preparation time: 15 minutes
Cooking time: 0 minutes
Servings: 4

Ingredients:

- ½ cup chopped walnuts
- Salt and black pepper to the taste
- 1 teaspoon lemon zest
- A pinch of chili flakes
- ¼ cup lemon juice
- 1 pound asparagus, trimmed and cut into medium pieces
- ¼ cup mint leaves
- A drizzle of olive oil

Directions:

In a bowl, mix together the walnuts, lemon zest, salt, pepper and chili flakes. Add the asparagus to the walnut mix and toss. Add the lemon juice, mint and oil as well then toss to coat and serve. Enjoy!

Nutrition: calories 100, fat 1, fiber 6, carbs 8, protein 6

Napa Cabbage Side Salad

Preparation time: 10 minutes
Cooking time: 0 minutes
Servings: 4

Ingredients:

- ½ cup red bell pepper, cut into thin strips
- 1 carrot, grated
- 4 cups napa cabbage, shredded
- 3 green onions, chopped
- 1 tablespoon sesame oil
- 2 teaspoons fresh grated ginger
- ½ teaspoon red pepper flakes, crushed
- 3 tablespoons balsamic vinegar
- 1 tablespoon coconut aminos

Directions:

In a salad bowl, mix the bell pepper with carrot, cabbage, green onions, oil, ginger, pepper flakes, vinegar and aminos. Toss and serve as a side dish.
Enjoy!

Nutrition: calories 160, fat 10, fiber 3, carbs 10, protein 5

Cabbage and Almond Salad

Preparation time: 10 minutes
Cooking time: 0 minutes
Servings: 4

Ingredients:
- 1 Napa cabbage, shredded
- 1 cup chopped almonds
- 1 bunch green onions, chopped
- ¼ cup blueberries
- ¼ cup balsamic vinegar
- 2 tablespoons coconut aminos
- ½ cup olive oil
- ¼ teaspoon fresh grated ginger
- A pinch of black pepper

Directions:
In a salad bowl, mix the cabbage with the almonds, green onions, blueberries, vinegar, coconut aminos, oil, ginger and black pepper. Mix well and serve as a side dish.
Enjoy!

Nutrition: calories 140, fat 3, fiber 3, carbs 8, protein 6

Cabbage and Scallions Salad

Preparation time: 10 minutes
Cooking time: 0 minutes
Servings: 4

Ingredients:
- 3 scallions, chopped
- 1 green cabbage head, shredded
- 1 red bell pepper, halved and cut into thin strips
- 2 carrots, chopped
- ½ cup chopped cilantro
- 3 tablespoons sunflower seeds
- 2 tablespoons sesame seeds
- ¼ cup balsamic vinegar
- 3½ tablespoons olive oil
- 1 tablespoon maple syrup

Directions:
In a salad bowl, mix the cabbage with the scallions, bell pepper, carrots, cilantro, vinegar, oil, maple syrup, sunflower and sesame seeds. Toss everything together well and serve as a side dish.
Enjoy!

Nutrition: calories 140, fat 4, fiber 3, carbs 5, protein 6

Celery and Raisin Salad

Preparation time: 10 minutes
Cooking time: 0 minutes
Servings: 4

Ingredients:
- ½ cup raisins
- 4 cups sliced celery
- ¼ cup chopped parsley
- ½ cup chopped walnuts
- Juice of ½ lemon
- 2 tablespoons olive oil
- Salt and black pepper to the taste

Directions:
In a salad bowl, mix celery with raisins, walnuts and parsley and stir. Add lemon juice, oil, salt and pepper, toss to coat and serve as a side dish.
Enjoy!

Nutrition: calories 120, fat 1, fiber 2, carbs 3, protein 5

Cumin Carrots

Preparation time: 10 minutes
Cooking time: 40 minutes
Servings: 4

Ingredients:
- 8 carrots, peeled
- 1 teaspoon cumin, ground
- A pinch of salt and black pepper
- 1 teaspoon dried thyme
- 3 tablespoons tahini
- 2½ tablespoons water
- ¼ tablespoon apple vinegar
- 1 tablespoon coconut aminos
- 1 teaspoon ground turmeric

Directions:
Spread the carrots on a lined baking sheet, add cumin, salt, pepper, thyme and the oil. Toss well then bake in the oven at 360 degrees F for 40 minutes. In a small bowl whisk the tahini with the water, apple vinegar, coconut aminos and turmeric. Divide the carrots between plates, spread the tahini mix all over and serve as a side dish.
Enjoy!

Nutrition: calories 181, fat 9, fiber 6, carbs 24, protein 7

Baked Green Beans

Preparation time: 10 minutes
Cooking time: 30 minutes
Servings: 4

Ingredients:

- 2 pounds green beans, trimmed
- A drizzle of olive oil
- 2 garlic cloves, minced
- 2 teaspoons lemon zest
- ½ cup coconut cream
- A pinch of red pepper flakes
- A pinch of salt and black pepper

Directions:
Grease a baking dish with the olive oil and add the green beans, lemon zest, coconut cream, pepper flakes, salt and pepper. Toss a bit then bake in the oven at 400 degrees F for 30 minutes. Divide between plates and serve.
Enjoy!

Nutrition: calories 200, fat 4, fiber 4, carbs 11, protein 7

Easy Green Bean Casserole

Preparation time: 10 minutes
Cooking time: 30 minutes
Servings: 6

Ingredients:

- 28 ounces canned green beans, drained
- ¼ cup almond milk
- A pinch of salt and black pepper
- 10 ounces coconut cream

Directions:
In a baking dish, combine the green beans with the almond milk, salt, pepper and cream. Toss a bit and bake in the oven at 350 degrees F for 30 minutes. Divide between plates and serve as a side dish.
Enjoy!

Nutrition: calories 121, fat 3, fiber 4, carbs 10, protein 3

Roasted Cauliflower

Preparation time: 10 minutes
Cooking time: 1 hour
Servings: 6

Ingredients:
- 1 cauliflower head, florets separated
- 1 red onion, cut into wedges
- 2 cups chopped tomatoes
- ½ pound green beans, trimmed
- A pinch of salt and black pepper
- 3 tablespoons olive oil
- 1 cup balsamic vinegar
- 2 tablespoon chopped parsley

Directions:
In a baking dish, mix the cauliflower with the onion, tomatoes, green beans, salt, pepper, oil and vinegar. Bake in the oven at 400 degrees F for 1 hour then divide between plates, sprinkle the parsley on top and serve.
Enjoy!

Nutrition: calories 162, fat 4, fiber 9, carbs 11, protein 7

Roasted Vegetables

Preparation time: 10 minutes
Cooking time: 25 minutes
Servings: 4

Ingredients:
- ¾ pound Brussels sprouts, halved
- 2 carrots, sliced
- A drizzle of olive oil
- 1 teaspoon chopped rosemary
- 1 tablespoon balsamic vinegar
- 1 teaspoon chopped thyme
- ½ cup cranberries, dried
- ½ cup chopped walnuts

Directions:
In a baking dish, mix the Brussels sprouts with the carrots, rosemary, oil, vinegar, thyme, cranberries and walnuts. Place in the oven and bake at 400 degrees F for 25 minutes.Divide between plates and serve as a side dish.
Enjoy!

Nutrition: calories 191, fat 5, fiber 8, carbs 13, protein 7

Creamy Corn

Preparation time: 10 minutes
Cooking time: 2 hours
Servings: 4

Ingredients:

- 40 ounces canned corn, drained
- 1 cup coconut milk, unsweetened
- A pinch of salt and black pepper
- 2 tablespoons chopped green onions

Directions:

In your slow cooker, mix the corn with the coconut milk, salt, pepper and green onions. Cover and cook on High for 2 hours then divide between plates and serve as a side dish.
Enjoy!

Nutrition: calories 132, fat 4, fiber 4, carbs 6, protein 4

Squash and Spinach

Preparation time: 10 minutes
Cooking time: 25 minutes
Servings: 4

Ingredients:

- 1 butternut squash, peeled and cubed
- 1 tablespoon olive oil
- A pinch of salt and black pepper
- 1 shallot, chopped
- ¼ cup red vinegar
- 7 cups baby spinach
- ½ cup chopped pecans, toasted

Directions:

Arrange the squash cubes on a lined baking sheet, drizzle with half of the oil, add salt and pepper and toss a little bit. Bake in the oven at 425 degrees F for 25 minutes. Then, in a salad bowl, mix the cooked and cooled squash with shallot, vinegar, spinach, pecans and the rest of the oil and serve.
Enjoy!

Nutrition: calories 307, fat 6, fiber 4, carbs 9, protein 6

Easy Acorn Squash Side Dish

Preparation time: 10 minutes
Cooking time: 50 minutes
Servings: 4

Ingredients:

- 4 acorn squash, quartered
- 3 tablespoons ground cinnamon
- ¼ cup coconut oil, melted

Directions:
Arrange the squash quarters on a lined baking sheet, drizzle with the coconut oil, sprinkle with the cinnamon and bake in the oven at 360 degrees F for 50 minutes. Divide between plates and serve as a side dish.
Enjoy!

Nutrition: calories 305, fat 14, fiber 9, carbs 49, protein 4

Easy Tomato Chickpea Salad

Preparation time: 10 minutes
Cooking time: 6 minutes
Servings: 4

Ingredients:

- 2 tablespoons olive oil
- 15 ounces canned chickpeas, drained and rinsed
- 2 pints cherry tomatoes, halved
- 2 teaspoons ground cumin
- ¼ cup chopped parsley
- A pinch of salt and black pepper

For the vinaigrette:

- 2 tablespoons olive oil
- 1 teaspoon minced shallot
- 1 tablespoon sherry vinegar

Directions:
Heat up a pan with 2 tablespoons oil over medium-high heat and add the chickpeas. Spread the chickpeas evenly in the pan and cook for 4 minutes. Add the cumin, salt and pepper and toss a bit then cook for 2 minutes more. Remove from heat and cool down then transfer to a bowl. Add the tomatoes and the parsley and toss. In another bowl, whisk together the 2 tablespoons oil with shallot and vinegar and pour over the salad. Toss well and serve as a side dish.
Enjoy!

Nutrition: calories 168, fat 9, fiber 3, carbs 8, protein 5

Fresh Green Beans

Preparation time: 10 minutes
Cooking time: 35 minutes
Servings: 6

Ingredients:

- 3 tablespoons olive oil
- 1 ½ cups chopped onion
- 1 tablespoon minced garlic
- A pinch of salt and black pepper
- 2 teaspoons garam masala
- 2 teaspoons fresh grated ginger
- ½ teaspoon ground cinnamon
- ½ teaspoon ground coriander
- 2 cups chopped tomatoes
- ½ cup vegetable stock
- ½ teaspoon brown mustard seeds
- 1½ pounds green beans, trimmed
- Juice of 1 lemon

Directions:
Heat up a large pan with the oil over medium-high heat and add the onion and the garlic. Stir and cook for 5 minutes. Add salt, pepper, garam masala, ginger, cinnamon, coriander, tomatoes, stock, mustard seeds and green beans. Mix well then reduce heat to medium-low and cook everything for 30 minutes. Add lemon juice, toss, divide between plates and serve.
Enjoy!

Nutrition: calories 181, fat 3, fiber 6, carbs 12, protein 6

Fast Tomato Side Salad

Preparation time: 10 minutes
Cooking time: 0 minutes
Servings: 4

Ingredients:

- 4 mixed colored tomatoes, chopped
- 1 cucumber, sliced
- A drizzle of olive oil
- 1 tablespoon chopped dill
- 1 red onion, chopped
- A pinch of salt and black pepper

Directions:
In a bowl, mix the tomatoes with the cucumber, onion, salt, pepper, dill and oil. Serve as a side dish.
Enjoy!

Nutrition: calories 171, fat 4, fiber 7, carbs 13, protein 6

Cabbage and Daikon Radish Mix

Preparation time: 10 minutes
Cooking time: 0 minutes
Servings: 6

Ingredients:
- 1 pound Napa cabbage, chopped
- 1 carrot, julienned
- A pinch of salt and black pepper
- ½ cup daikon radish
- 3 green onion stalks, chopped
- 3 tablespoons chili flakes
- 3 garlic cloves, minced
- 1 tablespoon sesame oil
- ½ inch fresh ginger, grated

Directions:
In a bowl, mix the cabbage with the carrot, daikon radish, onion, chili flakes, garlic, salt, pepper, ginger and oil. Toss well and serve as a side salad.
Enjoy!

Nutrition: calories 60, fat 3, fiber 2, carbs 5, protein 1

Minty Snap Peas

Preparation time: 10 minutes
Cooking time: 5 minutes
Servings: 4

Ingredients:
- ¾ pound sugar snap peas, trimmed
- Salt and black pepper to the taste
- 1 tablespoon chopped mint leaves
- 2 teaspoons olive oil
- 3 green onions, chopped
- 1 garlic clove, minced

Directions:
Heat up a pan with the oil over medium-high heat and add snap peas, salt, pepper, green onions, garlic and mint. Toss the mix well and then cook for 5 minutes. Divide between plates and serve as a side dish.
Enjoy!

Nutrition: calories 120, fat 6, fiber 1, carbs 5, protein 6

Collard Greens Mix

Preparation time: 10 minutes
Cooking time: 10 minutes
Servings: 4

Ingredients:

- 5 bunches collard greens, chopped
- Salt and black pepper to the taste
- 1 tablespoon crushed red pepper flakes
- 3 tablespoons chicken stock
- 2 tablespoons minced garlic
- ¼ cup olive oil

Directions:
Heat up a pot with the oil over medium heat and add the garlic. Stir and cook for 2 minutes. Add the collard greens, pepper flakes, stock, salt and pepper. Mix well and cook for 8 minutes then divide between plates and serve as a side dish.
Enjoy!

Nutrition: calories 212, fat 16, fiber 10, carbs 7, protein 6

Fast Swiss Chard

Preparation time: 10 minutes
Cooking time: 10 minutes
Servings: 4

Ingredients:

- 2 tablespoons olive oil
- 2 bunches Swiss chard, roughly chopped
- ½ teaspoon garlic paste
- 3 tablespoons lemon juice
- Salt and black pepper to the taste

Directions:
Heat a pan with the olive oil over medium heat and add the garlic paste. Stir and cook for 1 minute. Add Swiss chard, lemon juice, salt and pepper. Toss and cook for 8-9 minutes then divide between plates and serve as a side dish.
Enjoy!

Nutrition: calories 69, fat 7, fiber 1, carbs 2, protein 1

Watercress Side Salad

Preparation time: 10 minutes
Cooking time: 0 minutes
Servings: 4

Ingredients:

- 4 medium endives, trimmed and thinly sliced
- 1 tablespoon lemon juice
- 1 shallot, finely chopped
- 1 tablespoon balsamic vinegar
- 2 tablespoons olive oil
- 6 tablespoons coconut cream
- Salt and black pepper to the taste
- 4 ounces watercress, cut into medium springs
- 1 tablespoon chopped chervil
- 1 tablespoon chopped tarragon
- 1 tablespoon chopped chives
- 1/3 cup chopped almonds
- 1 tablespoon chopped parsley

Directions:

In a small bowl, whisk together the lemon juice with vinegar, salt, pepper, oil and shallot then set aside for 10 minutes. In a separate salad bowl, mix the endives with watercress, chives, tarragon, parsley, chervil, cream and the lemon juice mix. Toss and serve as a side dish with almonds sprinkled on top.
Enjoy!

Nutrition: calories 142, fat 3, fiber 5, carbs 4, protein 7

Zucchini and Carrot Mix

Preparation time: 15 minutes
Cooking time: 0 minutes
Servings: 6

Ingredients:

- 3 carrots, grated
- 2 zucchinis, sliced
- A bunch of radishes, sliced
- ½ red onion, chopped
- 6 mint leaves, roughly chopped

For the salad dressing:

- 1 teaspoon mustard
- 1 tablespoons balsamic vinegar
- 2 tablespoons olive oil
- A pinch of salt and black pepper

Directions:

In a bowl, mix the carrots with the radishes, zucchinis, onion and mint. In another bowl, whisk together the mustard with the vinegar, oil, salt and pepper. Add the dressing to the salad, toss and serve as a side dish.
Enjoy!

Nutrition: calories 117, fat 7, fiber 3, carbs 13, protein 1

Chili Eggplant Mix

Preparation time: 10 minutes
Cooking time: 15 minutes
Servings: 4

Ingredients:
- 1 big Asian eggplant, cubed
- 1 yellow onion, thinly sliced
- 2 tablespoon olive oil
- 2 teaspoons minced garlic
- 2 teaspoons chili paste
- ¼ cup coconut cream
- 4 green onions, chopped

Directions:
Heat up a pan with the oil over medium-high heat then add the onion, stir and cook for 3-4 minutes. Add the garlic, chili paste, green onions and coconut cream and stir, cooking for 2-3 minutes more. Add the eggplant, toss and cook for 7-8 minutes more. Divide between plates and serve as a side dish.
Enjoy!

Nutrition: calories 142, fat 7, fiber 4, carbs 5, protein 3

Spanish Spinach Mix

Preparation time: 10 minutes
Cooking time: 12 minutes
Servings: 4

Ingredients:
- 1 apple, cored and chopped
- 1 yellow onion, sliced
- 3 tablespoons olive oil
- 6 garlic cloves, chopped
- ¼ cup pine nuts, toasted
- ¼ cup balsamic vinegar
- 5 cups mixed spinach and Swiss chard
- Salt and black pepper to the taste
- A pinch of ground nutmeg

Directions:
Heat up a pan with the oil over medium-high heat, add onion, stir and cook for 3 minutes. Add apple, garlic, vinegar and spinach chard mix. Stir and cook for 10 minutes over medium-low heat. Add nutmeg, salt and pepper and toss. Divide between plates and serve.
Enjoy!

Nutrition: calories 120, fat 1, fiber 2, carbs 3, protein 6

Snack and Appetizer Recipes

Cumin Zucchini Slices

Preparation time: 10 minutes
Cooking time: 15 minutes
Servings: 4

Ingredients:
- ¼ cup tomato sauce
- 1 zucchini, sliced
- Salt and black pepper to the taste
- ½ teaspoon ground cumin
- Cooking spray

Directions:
Spray a baking sheet with cooking spray and spread the zucchini slices on the tray evenly. Pour the tomato sauce over the zucchini. Sprinkle with cumin, salt and pepper, introduce in the oven at 350 degrees F, bake for 15 minutes, arrange on a platter and serve.
Enjoy!

Nutrition: calories 140, fat 4, fiber 2, carbs 6, protein 4

Balsamic Zucchini Snack

Preparation time: 10 minutes
Cooking time: 3 hours
Servings: 8

Ingredients:
- 3 zucchinis, thinly sliced
- Salt and black pepper to the taste
- 2 tablespoons avocado oil
- 2 tablespoons balsamic vinegar

Directions:
In a bowl, whisk the oil with the vinegar, salt and pepper. Add zucchini slices to the bowl and toss to coat well. Spread the zucchini on a lined baking sheet and place the tray in the oven at 200 degrees F and bake for 3 hours. Leave chips to cool down and serve them.
Enjoy!

Nutrition: calories 100, fat 3, fiber 7, carbs 3, protein 7

Zucchini Spread

Preparation time: 10 minutes
Cooking time: 0 minutes
Servings: 5

Ingredients:
- 4 cups chopped zucchini
- ¼ cup olive oil
- Salt and black pepper to the taste
- 4 garlic cloves, minced
- ¾ cup tahini
- ½ cup lemon juice
- 1 tablespoon ground cumin

Directions:
In your blender, mix zucchini with salt, pepper, oil, lemon juice, garlic, tahini and cumin. Pulse until smooth then divide into small bowls and serve.
Enjoy!

Nutrition: calories 110, fat 5, fiber 3, carbs 6, protein 7

Celery Spread

Preparation time: 10 minutes
Cooking time: 0 minutes
Servings: 2

Ingredients:
- 6 celery stacks, chopped
- 3 tablespoons tomato sauce
- ¼ cup avocado mayonnaise
- Salt and black pepper to the taste
- ½ teaspoon garlic powder

Directions:
In a bowl, mix the celery with mayo, tomato sauce, black pepper, salt and garlic powder. Stir well and divide into bowls and serve.
Enjoy!

Nutrition: calories 100, fat 12, fiber 3, carbs 1, protein 6

Mushrooms Stuffed with Shrimp

Preparation time: 10 minutes
Cooking time: 20 minutes
Servings: 5

Ingredients:

- ¼ cup avocado mayonnaise
- 1 teaspoon garlic powder
- 1 small yellow onion, chopped
- 24 ounces white mushroom caps
- Salt and black pepper to the taste
- 1 teaspoon curry powder
- ¼ cup coconut cream
- 1 cup shrimp, cooked, peeled, deveined and chopped

Directions:

In a bowl, whisk together the mayo with garlic powder, onion, salt, pepper, curry powder, coconut cream and shrimp. Stuff the mushrooms with this mix and arrange them on a baking sheet. Cook in the oven at 350 degrees F for 20 minutes. Arrange on a platter and serve. Enjoy!

Nutrition: calories 204, fat 10, fiber 3, carbs 7, protein 11

Mango Salsa

Preparation time: 10 minutes
Cooking time: 0 minutes
Servings: 4

Ingredients:

- 1 avocado, pitted, peeled and cubed
- 2 cups cubed mango
- ¼ cup chopped cilantro
- ½ cup chopped red onion
- 2 tablespoons olive oil
- Salt and black pepper to the taste
- Juice of 1 lime
- A pinch of red pepper flakes

Directions:

In a bowl, mix avocado with mango, onion and cilantro. Add olive oil, salt, pepper, lime juice and pepper flakes then toss to coat and serve as a snack.
Enjoy!

Nutrition: calories 100, fat 3, fiber 4, carbs 8, protein 9

Kale Chips

Preparation time: 10 minutes
Cooking time: 1 hour and 30 minutes
Servings: 10

Ingredients:

- 2 cups cashews, soaked and drained
- 1 bunch kale, trimmed and leaves separated
- Salt and black pepper to the taste
- 3 tablespoons avocado oil
- Juice of 1 lemon
- 2/3 cup jarred roasted peppers
- 1 teaspoon Italian seasoning
- ¼ teaspoon chili powder
- ½ teaspoon garlic powder

Directions:
In your food processor, mix cashews with peppers, oil, lemon juice, Italian seasoning, chili power, garlic powder, salt and pepper and blend very well. In a bowl, mix kale leaves with cashews mix and massage well. Spread them on a lined baking sheet and bake in the oven at 400 degrees F for 1 hour. Flip and cook kale chips for 30 minutes more then allow to cool. Serve the chips cold
Enjoy!

Nutrition: calories 126, fat 7, fiber 2, carbs 9, protein 7

Green Bean Snack

Preparation time: 10 minutes
Cooking time: 8 hours
Servings: 8

Ingredients:

- 1/3 cup coconut oil, melted
- 5 pounds green beans
- Salt to the taste
- 1 teaspoon garlic powder
- 1 teaspoon onion powder

Directions:
In a bowl, mix green beans with coconut oil, salt, garlic and onion powder. Put them in your dehydrator and dry them for 8 hours at 135 degrees. Serve cold as a snack.
Enjoy!

Nutrition: calories 100, fat 12, fiber 4, carbs 8, protein 5

Avocado Hummus

Preparation time: 10 minutes
Cooking time: 0 minutes
Servings: 6

Ingredients:

- 2 avocados, peeled, pitted, chopped
- Salt and black pepper to the taste
- 1 tablespoon coconut oil
- 4 garlic cloves, chopped
- ½ cup tahini
- 2 tablespoons lemon juice
- 4 ounces roasted peppers, chopped

Directions:
In a blender, mix the avocados with salt, pepper, oil, garlic, tahini, lemon juice and peppers. Pulse until smooth then divide into bowls and serve as a snack.
Enjoy!

Nutrition: calories 140, fat 6, fiber 2, carbs 9, protein 8

Veggie Stuffed Mushrooms

Preparation time: 10 minutes
Cooking time: 30 minutes
Servings: 12

Ingredients:

- 1 tablespoon olive oil
- 2 small red bell peppers, chopped
- 1 small yellow onion, chopped
- 2 pounds button mushrooms, stems reserved
- 3 garlic cloves, minced
- 2 cups chopped spinach
- Salt and black pepper to the taste
- ¼ cup chopped parsley

Directions:
Heat up a pan with the oil over medium heat and add the mushroom stems. Stir and cook for 2 minutes. Add bell peppers, garlic, parsley, spinach, salt, pepper and onion. Stir, cook for 6 minutes then remove from heat. Stuff each mushroom with this mix and arrange them all on a lined baking sheet. Cook in the oven at 350 degrees F for 20 minutes and serve as an appetizer.
Enjoy!

Nutrition: calories 120, fat 8, fiber 5, carbs 10, protein 9

Sesame Spread

Preparation time: 10 minutes
Cooking time: 0 minutes
Servings: 6

Ingredients:
- 1 cup tahini sesame seed paste
- Salt and black pepper to the taste
- 1 cup veggie stock
- ½ cup lemon juice
- 1 tablespoon chopped cilantro
- ½ teaspoon ground cumin
- 3 garlic cloves, chopped

Directions:
Place the sesame seed paste with salt, pepper, lemon juice, stock, cilantro, cumin and garlic into a food processor. Pulse well, divide into bowls and serve as a party spread.
Enjoy!

Nutrition: calories 120, fat 12, fiber 2, carbs 11, protein 5

Eggplant Spread

Preparation time: 10 minutes
Cooking time: 0 minutes
Servings: 6

Ingredients:
- 2 pounds eggplant, baked, peeled and chopped
- A pinch of salt and black pepper
- 4 tablespoons olive oil
- 4 garlic cloves, chopped
- Juice of 1 lemon
- ¼ cup black olives, pitted
- 1 tablespoon sesame paste

Directions:
In a blender, mix the eggplant with salt, pepper, oil, garlic, lemon juice, olives and sesame paste. Blend until smooth then divide into bowls and serve.
Enjoy!

Nutrition: calories 165, fat 11, fiber 4, carbs 8, protein 5

Artichoke Spread

Preparation time: 10 minutes
Cooking time: 35 minutes
Servings: 6

Ingredients:
- 2 garlic cloves, minced
- Juice of ½ lemon
- 1 cup veggie stock
- 1 pound baby artichokes, trimmed and stems cut off
- 1 cup coconut cream
- A pinch of salt and black pepper

Directions:
In a small pot, mix the artichokes with the stock, salt and pepper. Stir and bring to a simmer over medium heat. Simmer for 35 minutes then transfer to a blender, add the garlic, lemon juice and cream and pulse well. Divide into bowls and serve.
Enjoy!

Nutrition: calories 150, fat 2, fiber 3, carbs 8, protein 5

Balsamic Onion Snack

Preparation time: 10 minutes
Cooking time: 10 minutes
Servings: 4

Ingredients:
- 1 pound pearl onions, peeled
- A pinch of salt and black pepper
- ½ cup water
- 4 tablespoons balsamic vinegar
- 1 tablespoon coconut flour

Directions:
In a small pot, whisk the water with the vinegar and coconut flour. Bring to a simmer over medium heat. Add the pearl onions, toss, cook for 10 minutes, Drain the liquid, divide into bowls and serve as a snack.
Enjoy!

Nutrition: calories 100, fat 9, fiber 4, carbs 11, protein 6

Lentil Cakes

Preparation time: 10 minutes
Cooking time: 10 minutes
Servings: 8

Ingredients:

- 2 teaspoons fresh grated ginger
- 1 cup chopped yellow onion
- 1 cup minced mushrooms
- 1 cup canned red lentils, drained and rinsed
- 1 sweet potato, grated
- ¼ cup chopped parsley
- 1 tablespoon curry powder
- ¼ cup chopped cilantro
- 2 tablespoons coconut flour
- 1 tablespoon olive oil

Directions:
Put the lentils in a bowl and mash them well using a potato masher. Add the onion, ginger, mushrooms, potato, curry powder, parsley, cilantro and the flour to the bowl with the lentils. Stir well and shape medium cakes out of this mix. Heat up a pan with the oil over medium-high heat, add the cakes and cook them for about 5 minutes on each side. Serve as an appetizer while warm. Enjoy!

Nutrition: calories 142, fat 4, fiber 3, carbs 8, protein 8

Tomato Salsa

Preparation time: 10 minutes
Cooking time: 0 minutes
Servings: 6

Ingredients:

- 3 cups chopped tomatoes
- 2 teaspoons capers
- 3 garlic cloves, minced
- 2 teaspoons balsamic vinegar
- 1 tablespoon chopped basil
- A pinch of salt and black pepper

Directions:
In a bowl, mix the tomatoes with the capers, garlic, vinegar, basil, salt and pepper. Toss the mix well then divide into smaller bowls and serve as an appetizer.
Enjoy!

Nutrition: calories 121, fat 3, fiber 1, carbs 8, protein 6

Pecan and Pea Spread

Preparation time: 10 minutes
Cooking time: 0 minutes
Servings: 8

Ingredients:

- ½ cup chopped pecans, toasted
- 1½ cups canned black-eyed peas, drained and rinsed
- ½ teaspoon chili powder
- A pinch of salt and black pepper
- ½ teaspoon garlic powder
- 1 teaspoon Cajun seasoning
- ½ teaspoon Tabasco sauce

Directions:

In a blender, mix the peas with the pecans, chili powder, salt, pepper, garlic powder, Cajun seasoning and Tabasco sauce. Pulse well, divide into bowls and serve as a party spread.
Enjoy!

Nutrition: calories 127, fat 5, fiber 7, carbs 18, protein 8

Easy Squash Spread

Preparation time: 10 minutes
Cooking time: 35 minutes
Servings: 8

Ingredients:

- ½ cup veggie stock
- ½ cup cubed butternut squash
- ½ cup white beans, soaked for 12 hours and drained
- 1 tablespoon olive oil
- 1 teaspoon ground sage
- 1 teaspoon rosemary, dried
- A pinch of salt and black pepper

Directions:

In a small pot, mix squash, beans and stock. Bring to a simmer over medium-high heat, cook for 35 minutes, drain and transfer the whole mixture to a blender. Add oil, sage, salt, pepper and rosemary then pulse really well. Divide into bowls and serve.
Enjoy!

Nutrition: calories 112, fat 5, fiber 2, carbs 8, protein 7

Cauliflower Spread

Preparation time: 10 minutes
Cooking time: 15 minutes
Servings: 4

Ingredients:
- 4 cups cauliflower florets
- 1½ cups chopped carrot
- 2 cups water
- ½ cup cashews
- A pinch of salt and black pepper
- 1 teaspoon smoked paprika
- ½ teaspoon chili powder
- ¼ teaspoon ground mustard
- ½ teaspoon ground jalapeno
- ½ cup chopped cilantro

Directions:
In a small pot, mix cauliflower with carrots, water and cashews. Stir the mix and bring to a boil over medium heat then cook for 15 minutes and strain into a blender. Add salt, pepper, paprika, chili powder, mustard powder, jalapeno powder and cilantro to the blender as well. Pulse, divide into bowls and serve.
Enjoy!

Nutrition: calories 130, fat 4, fiber 3, carbs 6, protein 7

Chard and Sesame Spread

Preparation time: 10 minutes
Cooking time: 10 minutes
Servings: 4

Ingredients:
- 2 garlic cloves, minced
- 2 cups Swiss chard leaves
- ½ cup veggie stock
- ¼ cup sesame paste
- 1 tablespoon chopped cilantro
- A pinch of salt and black pepper
- 2 teaspoons olive oil
- Juice of 1 lime

Directions:
Put the stock in a small pot and bring to a simmer over medium heat. Add the Swiss chard, salt and pepper to the pot, bring to a simmer and cook for about 10 minutes. Drain and put in a food processor along with the garlic, sesame paste, lime juice, olive oil and cilantro. Pulse well, divide into bowls and serve.
Enjoy!

Nutrition: calories 142, fat 6, fiber 3, carbs 7, protein 4

Peanut Butter Dip

Preparation time: 10 minutes
Cooking time: 0 minutes
Servings: 4

Ingredients:
- ½ cup coconut cream
- ¼ cup peanut butter, soft

Directions:
In a bowl, whisk together the peanut butter with the coconut cream. Divide into bowls and serve.
Enjoy!

Nutrition: calories 110, fat 1, fiber 5, carbs 7, protein 5

Snow Pea Salsa

Preparation time: 10 minutes
Cooking time: 0 minutes
Servings: 4

Ingredients:
- 1 avocado, peeled, pitted and roughly chopped
- 1½ cups snow peas, steamed and cooled
- 1 tablespoon lime juice
- 1 garlic clove, chopped
- A pinch of cayenne pepper

Directions:
In a bowl, mix the snow peas with the avocado, lime juice, garlic and cayenne pepper. Toss everything together well and serve.
Enjoy!

Nutrition: calories 120, fat 10, fiber 4, carbs 6, protein 6

Nutmeg Apple Snack

Preparation time: 10 minutes
Cooking time: 2 hours
Servings: 4

Ingredients:

- Cooking spray
- Ground Cinnamon to taste
- 2 apples, cored and cubed
- A pinch of ground nutmeg

Directions:
Arrange the apple cubes on a lined baking sheet and sprinkle with cinnamon, nutmeg and spray with the cooking oil. Toss the apples slices well and place in the oven at 275 degrees F. Bake for 2 hours.Divide into bowls and serve as a snack
Enjoy!

Nutrition: calories 141, fat 2, fiber 2, carbs 7, protein 5

Dill Coconut Dip

Preparation time: 10 minutes
Cooking time: 0 minutes
Servings: 4

Ingredients:

- 1½ cups coconut cream
- 2 teaspoons dried dill
- 2 teaspoons dried thyme
- 1 teaspoon sweet paprika
- 2 teaspoons sun-dried tomatoes, chopped
- 2 teaspoons dried parsley
- 2 teaspoons chopped chives
- A pinch of sea salt and black pepper

Directions:
In a bowl, mix the coconut cream with the dill, thyme, paprika, tomatoes, parsley, chives, salt and pepper and serve cold as a snack.
Enjoy!

Nutrition: calories 219, fat 20, fiber 0, carbs 5, protein 3

Sweet Potato Spread

Preparation time: 10 minutes
Cooking time: 15 minutes
Servings: 8

Ingredients:

- 1 cup canned garbanzo beans, drained and rinsed
- 4 cups chopped, peeled sweet potatoes
- ¼ cup sesame paste
- 2 tablespoons lime juice
- 1 tablespoon olive oil
- 5 garlic cloves, minced
- ½ teaspoon ground cumin
- 2 tablespoons water
- A pinch of salt

Directions:
Put the sweet potatoes in a steamer basket, add some water into a pot and place the basket on top. Bring to a boil over medium-high heat and steam potatoes for 15 minutes. Drain, let them cool and then put them into a blender. Add the sesame paste, garlic, beans, lemon juice, cumin, water, salt and oil. Pulse well, transfer to bowls and serve.
Enjoy!

Nutrition: calories 170, fat 3, fiber 7, carbs 10, protein 8

Dill Zucchini Patties

Preparation time: 10 minutes
Cooking time: 20 minutes
Servings: 12

Ingredients:

- Cooking spray
- ½ cup chopped dill
- 1 egg
- ½ cup coconut flour
- A pinch of sea salt and black pepper
- 1 yellow onion, chopped
- 2 garlic cloves, minced
- 3 zucchinis, grated and excess water squeezed

Directions:
In a bowl, mix zucchinis with garlic, onion, flour, salt, pepper, egg and dill. Shape medium patties out of this mix and arrange them on a lined baking sheet. Spray them with cooking oil, and bake in the oven at 400 degrees F for 10 minutes on each side. Arrange the patties on a platter and serve as an appetizer.
Enjoy!

Nutrition: calories 120, fat 4, fiber 2, carbs 6, protein 6

Italian Cauliflower Crackers

Preparation time: 10 minutes
Cooking time: 40 minutes
Servings: 12

Ingredients:
- 1 big cauliflower head, florets separated
- ¼ cup egg whites
- 1 teaspoon Italian seasoning
- A pinch of sea salt and black pepper
- Black pepper to the taste

Directions:
Put cauliflower florets in your food processor and pulse until you obtain your cauliflower "rice" then spread the rice on a lined baking sheet. Place in the oven at 375 degrees F, roast for 20 minutes then put in a clean bowl, squeezing to remove any excess moisture. Mix in salt, pepper, Italian seasoning and egg whites. Spread this into a lined rectangular pan and press well. Place in the oven at 375 degrees F and bake for 20 minutes. Cut into medium crackers and serve them cold.
Enjoy!

Nutrition: calories 120, fat 6, fiber 2, carbs 6, protein 7

Fast Baked Mushroom Caps

Preparation time: 10 minutes
Cooking time: 15 minutes
Servings: 2

Ingredients:
- 2 pound brown mushrooms, stems discarded
- A pinch of sea salt and black pepper
- Black pepper to the taste

Directions:
Arrange mushroom caps on a lined baking sheet, season them with a pinch of salt and black pepper and place in the oven at 400 degrees F. Bake for 15 minutes and divide into bowls to serve cold.
Enjoy!

Nutrition: calories 120, fat 2, fiber 8, carbs 6, protein 5

Almond Spinach Dip

Preparation time: 10 minutes
Cooking time: 35 minutes
Servings: 12

Ingredients:
- ½ cup almond milk
- 1½ cups coconut cream
- 10 ounces spinach
- 4 garlic cloves, minced
- ½ cup chopped green onions
- A pinch of black pepper
- 1 tablespoon oregano, dried
- Cooking spray

Directions:
In a bowl, mix the spinach with the almond milk, cream, garlic, green onions, oregano and black pepper. Spray a baking dish with cooking oil and spread the spinach dip in the pan, introduce in the oven at 350 degrees F and bake for 35 minutes. Leave your dip to cool down a bit before serving it.
Enjoy!

Nutrition: calories 130, fat 5, fiber 4, carbs 6, protein 6

Pineapple Salmon Bites

Preparation time: 10 minutes
Cooking time: 20 minutes
Servings: 2

Ingredients:
- 20 ounces canned pineapple pieces
- ½ teaspoon fresh grated ginger
- 2 teaspoons garlic powder
- 1 teaspoon onion powder
- 1 tablespoon balsamic vinegar
- 2 medium salmon fillets, boneless, skinless and cubed
- Black pepper to the taste

Directions:
Place salmon and pineapple pieces in a baking dish then add the ginger, garlic powder, onion powder, black pepper and vinegar. Toss the mix and place in the oven at 375 degrees F, bake for 20 minutes, divide into bowls and serve.
Enjoy!

Nutrition: calories 200, fat 3, fiber 3, carbs 7, protein 14

Parsley Shrimp Bowls

Preparation time: 10 minutes
Cooking time: 10 minutes
Servings: 2

Ingredients:

- 1 pound medium shrimp, peeled and deveined
- Juice of ½ lemon
- 1 pound asparagus, trimmed and chopped
- 2 teaspoons olive oil
- 4 garlic cloves, minced
- 1 small yellow onion, chopped
- 1 small parsley bunch, chopped
- A pinch of salt and black pepper

Directions:
Heat up a pan with the oil over medium-high heat, and then add onion and garlic. Stir and cook for 5 minutes. Add asparagus and shrimp, stir and cook for 4 minutes. Transfer this mix to a bowl and add salt, pepper, lemon juice and parsley. Toss the mix then divide into small bowls and serve.
Enjoy!

Nutrition: calories 135, fat 2, fiber 4, carbs 9, protein 12

Paprika Oysters

Preparation time: 10 minutes
Cooking time: 8 minutes
Servings: 3

Ingredients:

- 6 big oysters, shucked
- 3 garlic cloves, minced
- 1 lemon, cut into wedges
- 1 tablespoon parsley
- A pinch of sweet paprika
- 2 tablespoons coconut oil, melted

Directions:
Top each oyster with parsley and paprika then drizzle with the oil. Place them all on the preheated grill over medium-high heat and cook for 8 minutes. Serve oysters as an appetizer with lemon wedges on the side.
Enjoy!

Nutrition: calories 127, fat 13, fiber 0, carbs 5, protein 4

Dill Tuna Patties

Preparation time: 10 minutes
Cooking time: 10 minutes
Servings: 12

Ingredients:

- 15 ounces canned tuna, drain well and flaked
- 3 eggs
- 2 teaspoons chopped dill
- ½ cup chopped red onion
- 1 teaspoon garlic powder
- Salt and black pepper to the taste
- 2 tablespoons olive oil

Directions:

In a bowl, mix tuna with salt, pepper, dill, onion, garlic powder and eggs. Shape medium patties out of this mix. Heat up a pan with the oil over medium-high heat then add the patties, cook for 5 minutes on each side, arrange on a platter and serve while warm.
Enjoy!

Nutrition: calories 140, fat 2, fiber 5, carbs 7, protein 6

Lemony Shrimp Appetizer

Preparation time: 10 minutes
Cooking time: 6 minutes
Servings: 4

Ingredients:

- 2 tablespoons olive oil
- 1 pound shrimp, peeled and deveined
- 2 tablespoons lemon juice
- 2 tablespoons minced garlic
- 1 tablespoon lemon zest
- Salt and black pepper to the taste

Directions:

Heat up a pan with the oil over medium-high heat then add shrimp and cook for 2 minutes. Add garlic, lemon juice, lemon zest, salt and pepper. Stir and cook for 3-4 minutes more then divide into bowls and serve as an appetizer.
Enjoy!

Nutrition: calories 149, fat 6, fiber 3, carbs 9, protein 12

Shrimp and Snap Pea Salad

Preparation time: 10 minutes
Cooking time: 12 minutes
Servings: 4

Ingredients:

- 1 pound shrimp, peeled and deveined
- Salt and black pepper to the taste
- 4 cherry tomatoes, chopped
- 2 cups sugar snap peas, sliced lengthwise
- 1 red bell pepper, sliced
- 1 tablespoon olive oil
- ½ cup chopped cilantro
- 1 tablespoon minced garlic
- ½ cup chopped green onion
- ½ teaspoon red pepper flakes
- 10 ounces coconut milk
- 2 tablespoons lime juice

Directions:

Heat up a pan with the oil over medium-high heat and add snap peas then stir fry for 2 minutes. Add pepper, cilantro, garlic, green onions and pepper flakes. Stir and cook for 2 minutes. Add tomatoes and coconut milk then stir and simmer everything for 5 minutes. Add shrimp, salt, pepper and lime juice. Stir, cook for 3 minutes more. Divide into small bowls and serve as an appetizer.
Enjoy!

Nutrition: calories 150, fat 3, fiber 3, carbs 5, protein 7

Shrimp and Cucumber Noodle Salad

Preparation time: 10 minutes
Cooking time: 0 minutes
Servings: 4

Ingredients:

- 1 cucumber, cut with a spiralizer
- ½ cup chopped basil
- ½ pound shrimp, already cooked, peeled and deveined
- Salt and black pepper to the taste
- 2 tablespoons lime juice
- 2 teaspoons chili garlic sauce

Directions:

In a bowl, mix the cucumber with the basil, shrimp, salt, pepper, lime juice and chili sauce. Toss and serve as an appetizer.
Enjoy!

Nutrition: calories 130, fat 8, fiber 3, carbs 8, protein 8

Salmon Salsa

Preparation time: 10 minutes
Cooking time: 12 minutes
Servings: 2

Ingredients:

- 2 salmon fillets, boneless
- ½ cup chopped yellow onion
- 4 teaspoons olive oil
- 1 teaspoon Greek seasoning
- 1 teaspoon minced garlic
- 1 green bell pepper, chopped
- ½ cup canned tomato salsa
- 2 tablespoons kalamata olives, pitted and chopped
- ¼ cup vegetable stock
- Salt and black pepper to the taste

Directions:

Heat up a pan with half of the oil over medium heat, add bell pepper, garlic, Greek seasoning and onion, stir and cook for 5 minutes. Add stock, olives and salsa, toss, cook for 3-4 minutes more and transfer to the bowl. Heat up the same pan with the rest of the oil over medium heat, add fish, season with salt and pepper and cook for 2 minutes on each side, transfer to a cutting board, cut into medium cubes and put them in a baking dish. Add the salsa, toss, bake in the oven at 425 degrees F for 6 minutes, divide into bowls and serve cold as an appetizer. Enjoy!

Nutrition: calories 170, fat 5, fiber 2, carbs 7, protein 7

Creole Shrimp Platter

Preparation time: 10 minutes
Cooking time: 4 minutes
Servings: 2

Ingredients:

- ½ pound big shrimp, peeled and deveined
- 2 teaspoons olive oil
- Juice of 1 lime
- Salt and black pepper to the taste
- 1 teaspoon Creole seasoning

Directions:

Heat up a pan with the oil over medium-high heat, add the shrimp, lime juice, salt, pepper and Creole seasoning. Toss and cook the shrimp for 2 minutes on each side. Arrange the shrimp on a platter and serve as an appetizer. Enjoy!

Nutrition: calories 120, fat 3, fiber 5, carbs 8, protein 18

Mussels Bowls

Preparation time: 5 minutes
Cooking time: 5 minutes
Servings: 4

Ingredients:

- 2 pound mussels, debearded and scrubbed
- 2 garlic cloves, minced
- 1 tablespoon olive oil
- 1 tablespoon lemon juice

Directions:
Put some water in a pot, add the mussels, bring to a boil over medium heat, cook for 5 minutes and then discard unopened mussels. Transfer the cooked mussels to a bowl. Add olive oil, garlic and lemon juice then toss and serve as an appetizer.
Enjoy!

Nutrition: calories 90, fat 4, fiber 5, carbs 5, protein 14

Fried Squid

Preparation time: 10 minutes
Cooking time: 20 minutes
Servings: 2

Ingredients:

- 1 squid, cut into medium rings
- A pinch of cayenne pepper
- 1 egg, whisked
- 2 tablespoons coconut flour
- A pinch of salt and black pepper
- 2 tablespoons coconut oil
- 1 tablespoons lemon juice
- 4 tablespoons avocado mayonnaise
- 1 teaspoon sriracha sauce

Directions:
In a bowl, mix the squid rings with salt, pepper and cayenne. In another bowl, whisk the egg with salt, pepper and coconut flour. Dredge the squid rings in this mix. Heat up a pan with the oil over medium heat, add calamari rings and cook them for 5-6 minutes on each side then divide into bowls. In a small bowl, whisk the lemon juice with the mayo and the sriracha sauce and serve the rings with this mix.
Enjoy!

Nutrition: calories 155, fat 8, fiber 3, carbs 3, protein 7

Seafood Appetizer Bowls

Preparation time: 10 minutes
Cooking time: 15 minutes
Servings: 2

Ingredients:

- 8 ounces calamari, cut into medium rings
- 7 ounces shrimp, peeled and deveined
- 1 tablespoon coconut oil, melted
- 2 tablespoons avocado, chopped
- 1 teaspoon tomato paste
- 1 tablespoon mayonnaise
- 1 teaspoon lemon juice
- Salt and black pepper to the taste
- ½ teaspoon ground turmeric

Directions:

Grease a baking dish with the coconut oil, add calamari, shrimp, tomato paste, lemon juice, salt, pepper and turmeric. Toss and bake in the oven at 400 degrees F for 15 minutes. Remove from the oven, add the avocado, toss and divide into bowls and serve as an appetizer.
Enjoy!

Nutrition: calories 238, fat 8, fiber 3, carbs 10, protein 8

Celery Octopus Appetizer

Preparation time: 10 minutes
Cooking time: 40 minutes
Servings: 2

Ingredients:

- 21-ounces octopus, rinsed
- Juice of 1 lemon
- 4 celery stalks, chopped
- 3 ounces olive oil
- Salt and black pepper to the taste
- 4 tablespoons chopped parsley

Directions:

Put the octopus in a pot, add water to cover then cover the pot. Bring to a boil over medium heat and cook for 40 minutes. Drain, cool down the cooked octopus, chop and put in a salad bowl. Add celery stalks, parsley, oil, salt, pepper and lemon juice. Mix well, divide into small bowls and serve as an appetizer.
Enjoy!

Nutrition: calories 110, fat 6, fiber 3, carbs 6, protein 13

Coconut Cream Clams Mix

Preparation time: 10 minutes
Cooking time: 2 hours
Servings: 4

Ingredients:

- 1 cup chopped celery stalks
- Salt and black pepper to the taste
- 1 teaspoon ground thyme
- 2 cups vegetable stock
- A drizzle of olive oil
- 14 ounces canned baby clams
- 2 cups coconut cream
- 1 cup chopped onion

Directions:
Heat up a pan with the oil over medium heat and add the celery and onion. Stir and cook for 5 minutes. Transfer this mix to a crockpot and add the baby clams, salt, pepper, stock, thyme and cream. Stir and cook on High for 2 hours then divide into bowls and serve as an appetizer. Enjoy!

Nutrition: calories 220, fat 8, fiber 0, carbs 5, protein 12

Herbed Shrimp and Endive Salad

Preparation time: 10 minutes
Cooking time: 10 minutes
Servings: 4

Ingredients:

- 2 tablespoons olive oil
- 1 pound shrimp, peeled and deveined
- Salt and black pepper to the taste
- 2 tablespoons lime juice
- 3 endives, shredded
- 3 tablespoons chopped parsley
- 2 teaspoons chopped mint
- 1 tablespoon chopped tarragon
- 2 tablespoons mayonnaise
- 1 teaspoon lime zest

Directions:
In a bowl, mix shrimp with salt, pepper and the olive oil. Toss to coat then spread the shrimp on a lined baking sheet. Bake in the oven at 400 degrees F for 10 minutes. Remove from oven and the add lime juice, toss and transfer to a bowl. Add the endive, parsley, mint, tarragon, mayo, and lemon zest. Toss together and serve as an appetizer.
Enjoy!

Nutrition: calories 160, fat 7, fiber 2, carbs 7, protein 8

Citrus Oyster Platter

Preparation time: 10 minutes
Cooking time: 0 minutes
Servings: 4

Ingredients:

- 12 oysters, shucked
- Juice of 1 lemon
- Juice of 1 orange
- Zest of 1 orange
- Juice of 1 lime
- Zest of 1 lime
- 1 Serrano chili pepper, chopped
- 1 cup tomato juice
- ½ teaspoon fresh grated ginger
- ¼ teaspoon minced garlic
- A pinch of salt and black pepper
- ¼ cup olive oil
- ¼ cup chopped cilantro
- ¼ cup chopped scallions

Directions:
In a bowl, mix the lemon and the orange juice with lime zest, lime juice, orange zest, chili pepper, tomato juice, ginger, garlic, salt, pepper, oil, scallions and cilantro. Stir really well then spoon this mix into the oysters and serve them as an appetizer.
Enjoy!

Nutrition: calories 160, fat 8, fiber 6, carbs 16, protein 5

Asian Salmon Wraps

Preparation time: 10 minutes
Cooking time: 0 minutes
Servings: 12

Ingredients:

- 2 nori sheets
- 1 small avocado, pitted, peeled and chopped
- 6 ounces smoked salmon, sliced
- 4 ounces coconut cream
- 1 cucumber, sliced
- 1 teaspoon wasabi paste

Directions:
Place nori sheets on a sushi mat. Divide salmon slices, avocado and cucumber slices on each piece of nori. In a bowl, whisk together coconut cream with wasabi paste. Spread this over the cucumber and roll your nori sheets. Cut each into medium pieces and serve as an appetizer.
Enjoy!

Nutrition: calories 120, fat 6, fiber 6, carbs 12, protein 6

Mussels Appetizer

Preparation time: 10 minutes
Cooking time: 10 minutes
Servings: 6

Ingredients:

- 2 pounds mussels
- 2 ounces canned crushed tomatoes
- 2 ounces canned chopped tomatoes
- 2 tablespoons chicken soup
- 1 teaspoon crushed red pepper flakes
- 3 garlic cloves, minced
- 1 handful chopped parsley
- 1 yellow onion, chopped
- Salt and black pepper to the taste
- 1 tablespoon olive oil

Directions:

Heat up a Dutch oven over medium-high heat with the oil then add onion, stir and cook for 3 minutes. Add garlic, red pepper flakes, crushed and chopped tomatoes then stir. Add the stock, salt, pepper and the mussels then toss, cook for a few minutes until the mussels open. Discard unopened mussels then mix the opened mussels with the parsley. Toss the mix, divide into bowls and serve.
Enjoy!

Nutrition: calories 150, fat 3, fiber 3, carbs 6, protein 15

Sushi Appetizer

Preparation time: 10 minutes
Cooking time: 7 minutes
Servings: 4

Ingredients:

- 1 ahi tuna steak
- 2 tablespoons olive oil
- 1 cauliflower head, florets separated and riced
- 2 tablespoons green onions, chopped
- 1 avocado, pitted, peeled and chopped
- 1 cucumber, grated

For the salad dressing:

- 1 tablespoon sesame oil
- 2 tablespoons coconut aminos
- 1 tablespoon apple cider vinegar
- A pinch of salt

Directions:

Put some water in a pot, add a steamer basket inside, add cauliflower rice and bring to a boil over medium heat. Cover the pot, steam for a few minutes then drain and divide into bowls. Heat up a pan with the coconut oil over medium-high heat and add the tuna. Cook for 1 minute on each side and divide into the bowls with the rice. Also divide the green onions, cucumber and avocado among the bowls. In a separate small bowl, whisk together the sesame oil with the aminos, vinegar and a pinch of salt. Drizzle the dressing over the sushi bowls and serve as an appetizer.
Enjoy!

Nutrition: calories 210, fat 10, fiber 6, carbs 6, protein 12

Chicken Bites

Preparation time: 10 minutes
Cooking time: 10 minutes
Servings: 2

Ingredients:
- ½ cup almond flour
- 1 egg
- 2 tablespoons garlic powder
- 2 chicken breasts, cubed
- Salt and black pepper to the taste
- ½ cup coconut oil

Directions:
In a bowl, mix garlic powder with the flour, salt and pepper and stir. In another bowl, whisk the egg well. Dip the chicken breast pieces in the egg mix, then in flour mix. Heat up a pan with the oil over medium heat then drop chicken pieces into the hot pan. Cook them for 5 minutes on each side then divide into bowls and serve as a snack.
Enjoy!

Nutrition: calories 60, fat 3, fiber 2, carbs 6, protein 7

Meat Stuffed Mushrooms

Preparation time: 10 minutes
Cooking time: 10 minutes
Servings: 6

Ingredients:
- 16 ounces button mushroom caps
- 4 ounces coconut cream
- ¼ cup chopped carrot
- 4 tablespoons hot sauce
- ¼ cup chopped red onion
- ½ cup chicken meat, already cooked and chopped
- Salt and black pepper to the taste
- Cooking spray

Directions:
In a bowl, mix the cream with the carrot, hot sauce, onion, chicken, salt and pepper. Stuff the mushrooms with this mix and arrange them on a lined baking sheet. Spray with cooking spray and place in the oven at 425 degrees F. Bake for 10 minutes then arrange them on a platter and serve as an appetizer.
Enjoy!

Nutrition: calories 150, fat 4, fiber 6, carbs 14, protein 6

Stuffed Avocado

Preparation time: 10 minutes
Cooking time: 0 minutes
Servings: 2

Ingredients:

- 2 avocados, halved, pitted and flesh scooped out
- ¼ cup mayonnaise
- 1 teaspoon dried thyme
- 2 tablespoons coconut cream
- 1½ cups chicken, cooked and shredded
- Salt and black pepper to the taste
- ¼ teaspoon cayenne pepper
- ½ teaspoon onion powder
- ½ teaspoon garlic powder
- 1 teaspoon paprika
- Salt and black pepper to the taste
- 2 tablespoons lemon juice

Directions:
In a bowl, mash the avocado flesh with a fork. Add mayo, thyme, cream, chicken, salt, pepper, cayenne, onion powder, garlic powder, paprika, salt, pepper and lemon juice and mix well. Stuff the avocado skins with this mix, arrange them on a platter and serve as an appetizer.
Enjoy!

Nutrition: calories 160, fat 10, fiber 7, carbs 12, protein 7

Radish Chips

Preparation time: 10 minutes
Cooking time: 20 minutes
Servings: 4

Ingredients:

- Cooking spray
- 15 radishes, sliced
- Salt and black pepper to the taste
- 1 tablespoon chopped chives

Directions:
Arrange radish slices on a lined baking sheet, spray them with cooking oil, season with salt and pepper, sprinkle chives and place in the oven at 375 degrees F. Bake for 10 minutes on each side, divide into bowls and serve cold.
Enjoy!

Nutrition: calories 30, fat 1, fiber 2, carbs 7, protein 1

Avocado Appetizer Cream

Preparation time: 10 minutes
Cooking time: 10 minutes
Servings: 4

Ingredients:

- 2 avocados, pitted, peeled and chopped
- 3 cups chicken stock
- 2 scallions, chopped
- Salt and black pepper to the taste
- 2 tablespoons coconut oil
- 2/3 cup coconut cream, unsweetened

Directions:
Heat up a pot with the coconut oil over medium heat. Add scallions, stir and cook for 2 minutes. Add 2 ½ cups stock, stir and simmer for 3 minutes. In your blender, mix avocados with the rest of the stock, salt, pepper and cream. Pulse well and add this to the pot as well. Stir everything, cook for 2 minutes, divide into bowls and serve cold as an appetizer.
Enjoy!

Nutrition: calories 162, fat 8, fiber 4, carbs 6, protein 6

Tamarind Chutney

Preparation time: 10 minutes
Cooking time: 32 minutes
Servings: 10

Ingredients:

- 1 teaspoon cumin seeds
- 1 tablespoon coconut oil
- ½ teaspoon garam masala
- 1 teaspoon ground ginger
- ½ teaspoon fennel seeds
- ½ teaspoon cayenne pepper
- 2 cups water
- 3 tablespoons tamarind paste

Directions:
Heat up a pan with the oil over medium heat. Add the ginger, cumin, cayenne pepper, fennel seeds and garam masala to the heated pan. Stir and cook for 2 minutes. Add water and tamarind paste then stir, bring to a boil and reduce heat to low, simmering the chutney for 30 minutes. Transfer to bowls and leave the mix to cool down before you serve as an appetizer.
Enjoy!

Nutrition: calories 120, fat 1, fiber 3, carbs 5, protein 6

Pepper and Onion Appetizer

Preparation time: 10 minutes
Cooking time: 32 minutes
Servings: 4

Ingredients:

- 1 tablespoon olive oil
- 2 red bell peppers, cut into thin strips
- 2 red onions, cut into thin strips
-

- Salt and black pepper to the taste
- 1 teaspoon dried basil

Directions:

Heat up a pan with the oil over medium heat then add onion and bell peppers. Stir and cook for 2 minutes. Reduce temperature and cook for 30 minutes more stirring often. Add salt, pepper and basil, stir again, remove from heat and serve as a party dip.
Enjoy!

Nutrition: calories 107, fat 4, fiber 2, carbs 6, protein 6

Chia Crackers

Preparation time: 10 minutes
Cooking time: 35 minutes
Servings: 36

Ingredients:

- 1 cup ice water
- 1 cup ground chia seeds
- 2 tablespoons olive oil
- 2 tablespoons psyllium husk powder
- ¼ teaspoon dried oregano

- ¼ teaspoon garlic powder
- ¼ teaspoon onion powder
- Salt and black pepper to the taste
- ¼ teaspoon sweet paprika

Directions:

In a bowl, mix chia seeds with psyllium powder, oregano, garlic, onion powder, paprika, salt, pepper, oil and water. Stir until you obtain a firm mix then spread it on a baking sheet and place in the oven at 350 degrees F and bake for 35 minutes. Remove from the oven and set aside to cool down. Cut into medium crackers and serve as a snack.
Enjoy!

Nutrition: calories 50, fat 3, fiber 1, carbs 5, protein 2

Cilantro Guacamole

Preparation time: 3 hours
Cooking time: 0 minutes
Servings: 4

Ingredients:
- 2 avocados, pitted, peeled and chopped
- ½ cup chopped cilantro
- Juice and zest of 2 limes
- 1 cup coconut milk

Directions:
In a blender, mix the avocados with the coconut milk, cilantro, lime juice and zest. Pulse well, divide into bowls and serve as a snack.
Enjoy!

Nutrition: calories 150, fat 7, fiber 6, carbs 8, protein 4

Shrimp and Blackberries Bowls

Preparation time: 10 minutes
Cooking time: 5 minutes
Servings: 4

Ingredients:
- 2 tablespoons olive oil
- 1 pound shrimp, deveined and peeled
- 1 tablespoon chopped mint
- ½ cup blackberries
- 1 tablespoon balsamic vinegar

Directions:
Heat up a pan with the oil over medium-high heat, add the shrimp, toss and cook for 2 minutes on each side. Add the blackberries, mint and the vinegar. Mix and cook for 2-3 minutes more then divide into bowls and serve as an appetizer.
Enjoy!

Nutrition: calories 205, fat 9, fiber 3, carbs 8, protein 38

Jalapeno and Avocado Salsa

Preparation time: 10 minutes
Cooking time: 0 minutes
Servings: 4

Ingredients:
- 1 small red onion, chopped
- 2 avocados, pitted, peeled and chopped
- 3 jalapeno peppers, chopped
- Salt and black pepper to the taste
- 2 tablespoons cumin powder
- 2 tablespoons lime juice
- ½ tomato, chopped

Directions:
In a bowl, mix the onion with the avocados, jalapenos, salt, pepper, cumin, lime juice and tomato. Divide into smaller bowls and serve.
Enjoy!

Nutrition: calories 120, fat 2, fiber 2, carbs 7, protein 4

Easy Lime Crackers

Preparation time: 10 minutes
Cooking time: 20 minutes
Servings: 4

Ingredients:
- 1 cup almond flour
- Salt and black pepper to the taste
- 1½ teaspoons lime zest
- 1 teaspoon lime juice
- 1 egg

Directions:
In a bowl, whisk together the almond flour with lime zest, lime juice, salt and the egg. Divide this mix into 4 parts, roll each into a ball, and then spread it flat using a rolling pin. Cut each into 6 triangles, place them on a lined baking sheet and bake in the oven at 350 degrees F for 20 minutes.
Enjoy!

Nutrition: calories 58, fat 5, fiber 1, carbs 2, protein 3

Poultry Recipes

Chicken Soup

Preparation time: 10 minutes
Cooking time: 1 hour
Servings: 8

Ingredients:

- 2 tablespoons olive oil
- 2 celery stalks, chopped
- 2 carrots, chopped
- 1 yellow onion, chopped
- A pinch of salt and black pepper
- 5 garlic cloves, minced
- 8 cups chicken stock
- 2½ pounds chicken thighs, boneless and skinless
- 3 tablespoons chopped parsley
- 2 tablespoons lemon juice
- 2 tablespoons chopped dill

Directions:
Heat up a soup pot with the oil over medium-high heat. Add the celery, onion, carrots and garlic then stir and cook for 10 minutes. Add the chicken, stock, salt and pepper, stir then bring to a boil and reduce heat to medium-low. Cover and cook for 40 minutes. Transfer the chicken to a cutting board, shred the meat, discard bones and return the shredded chicken to the pot. Cook everything for a 4-5 minutes more, add parsley, dill and lemon juice then toss, ladle into bowls and serve.
Enjoy!

Nutrition: calories 211, fat 4, fiber 7, carbs 13, protein 8

Fruity Chicken Legs

Preparation time: 10 minutes
Cooking time: 8 hours
Servings: 4

Ingredients:

- Zest of 1 orange
- Juice of 1 orange
- ¼ cup red vinegar
- A pinch of salt and black pepper
- 4 chicken legs
- 5 garlic cloves, minced
- 1 red onion, cut into wedges
- 7 ounces canned peaches, halved
- ½ cup chopped parsley

Directions:
In a slow cooker, mix the orange zest with the orange juice, vinegar, salt, pepper, garlic, onion, peaches and parsley. Add the chicken, toss, cover and cook on Low for 8 hours. Divide between plates and serve.
Enjoy!

Nutrition: calories 251, fat 4, fiber 8, carbs 14, protein 8

Skillet Chicken Mix

Preparation time: 10 minutes
Cooking time: 15 minutes
Servings: 4

Ingredients:

- 1½ pounds chicken thighs, skinless and boneless
- 1 tablespoon olive oil
- 2 teaspoons chopped thyme
- A pinch of salt and black pepper
- 12 ounces Brussels sprouts, shredded
- 1 apple, cored and sliced
- ½ red onion, sliced
- 1 garlic clove, minced
- 2 tablespoons balsamic vinegar
- ¼ cup walnuts, chopped

Directions:

Heat up a pan with the oil over medium-high heat then add the chicken thighs, season with salt, pepper and thyme. Cook for 5 minutes on each side and transfer to a bowl. Heat up the pan again over medium heat, add the onion, apple, sprouts and garlic. Toss the mix and cook for 5 minutes. Add vinegar to the pan and return the chicken as well. Add the walnuts, toss, cook for 1-2 minutes more then divide between plates and serve.
Enjoy!

Nutrition: calories 211, fat 4, fiber 7, carbs 13, protein 8

Chicken Chili

Preparation time: 10 minutes
Cooking time: 20 minutes
Servings: 4

Ingredients:

- 1 pound ground chicken
- 1 cup chopped yellow onion
- 1½ tablespoons olive oil
- 2 garlic cloves, minced
- 30 ounces canned black beans, drained and rinsed
- 28 ounces roasted tomatoes, chopped
- 3 cups cubed butternut squash
- 14 ounces chicken stock
- A pinch of salt and black pepper

Directions:

Heat up a pot with the oil over medium-high heat, add the chicken, garlic and onion. Stir and cook for 6 minutes. Add the beans, tomatoes, squash, stock, salt and pepper. Stir the mix and bring to a simmer then cook over medium heat for 15 minutes. Divide into bowls and serve. Enjoy!

Nutrition: calories 211, fat 4, fiber 4, carbs 8, protein 7

Chipotle Chicken

Preparation time: 10 minutes
Cooking time: 12 minutes
Servings: 4

Ingredients:

- 1 pound chicken breasts, skinless, boneless and cut into strips
- 1 teaspoon chili powder
- 1 teaspoon ground cumin
- A pinch of salt and black pepper
- 1 tablespoon olive oil
- 1 red bell pepper, sliced
- 1 cup halved mushrooms
- 1 yellow onion, chopped
- 3 garlic cloves, minced
- 1 tablespoon chopped chipotles in adobo
- 1½ tablespoons lime juice

Directions:

Heat up a pan with the oil over medium-high heat and add the chicken. Mix and cook for 3-4 minutes. Add the chili powder, the cumin, salt, pepper, bell pepper, mushrooms, onion, garlic, chipotles and lime juice. Mix and cook for 7 minutes more, divide into bowls and serve.
Enjoy!

Nutrition: calories 241, fat 4, fiber 7, carbs 14, protein 7

Mexican Chicken Soup

Preparation time: 10 minutes
Cooking time: 8 hours
Servings: 4

Ingredients:

- 1 ¼ pounds chicken thighs, skinless and bone-in
- 1 yellow onion, chopped
- ½ red bell pepper, chopped
- 2 cups chicken stock
- 1 garlic clove, minced
- 14 ounces canned tomatoes, chopped
- 7 ounces tomato sauce
- 4 ounces canned green chilies, chopped
- 1 teaspoon dried oregano
- 1 teaspoon chili powder
- 1 teaspoon ground cumin
- A pinch of salt and black pepper
- 2 yellow squash, cubed
- 3 ounces green beans, halved
- 1 tablespoon lime juice
- 2½ tablespoons chopped cilantro

Directions:

In your slow cooker, mix the chicken with the onion, bell pepper, stock, garlic, tomatoes, tomato sauce, green chilies, oregano, chili powder, cumin, salt, pepper, squash, green beans and lime juice. Mix and cover then cook on Low for 8 hours. Once cooked, add the cilantro, stir, divide into bowls and serve.
Enjoy!

Nutrition: calories 261, fat 14, fiber 8, carbs 15, protein 10

Chicken and Barley Casserole

Preparation time: 10 minutes
Cooking time: 35 minutes
Servings: 4

Ingredients:

- 4 pounds chicken breasts, skinless and boneless
- A pinch of salt and black pepper
- A pinch of sweet paprika
- 3 tablespoons olive oil
- ¼ pounds mushrooms, sliced
- 1 cup barley
- 1 yellow onion, chopped
- 1 teaspoon dried basil
- 28 ounces chicken stock
- 8 ounces canned artichokes, drained and chopped
- 1 tablespoon chopped parsley

Directions:

Heat up a pan with half of the oil over medium-high heat. Add the chicken, season with salt and pepper and cook for 3-4 minutes on each side then transfer to a bowl. Heat up the same pan with the rest of the oil over medium-high heat then add mushrooms, onion and barley. Stir and cook for 7-8 minutes more. Add the stock and the basil, toss, bring to a boil, reduce heat to medium-low and simmer for 30 minutes. Return the chicken to the pan, cover and simmer everything for 20 minutes more. Add the artichoke hearts, simmer the mixture for 10 minutes more, divide between plates, sprinkle the parsley on top and serve.
Enjoy!

Nutrition: calories 312, fat 7, fiber 7, carbs 15, protein 15

Chicken Thighs and Chickpeas

Preparation time: 10 minutes
Cooking time: 40 minutes
Servings: 4

Ingredients:

- 8 chicken thighs, skin-on and bone-in
- 3 teaspoons olive oil
- 3 garlic cloves, minced
- A pinch of salt and black pepper
- 1 small yellow onion, chopped
- ½ teaspoon ground cumin
- 1 ½ teaspoon smoked paprika
- 1-pint grape tomatoes, halved
- 1 tablespoon chopped thyme
- 30 ounces canned chickpeas, drained and rinsed

Directions:

Heat up a pan with the olive oil over medium-high heat then add the chicken, season with salt and pepper and cook for 10 minutes. Once cooked, transfer to a plate. Add the garlic and the onion to the pan, stir and cook for 4 minutes. Mix in the cumin, paprika, chickpeas and tomatoes. Transfer the whole mixture to the oven and bake at 350 degrees F for 25 minutes. Sprinkle with the thyme, divide the mixture between plates and serve.
Enjoy!

Nutrition: calories 251, fat 4, fiber 7, carbs 13, protein 22

146

Chicken and Tasty Couscous

Preparation time: 10 minutes
Cooking time: 20 minutes
Servings: 4

Ingredients:
- 6 ounces couscous, cooked
- 2 teaspoon coconut oil
- 12 ounces baby carrots
- 4 chicken thighs, boneless
- A pinch of salt and black pepper
- 1/3 cup roasted pepitas
- 1/3 cup chopped parsley
- ¼ cup chopped mint
- 1 tablespoon olive oil
- 1 garlic clove, minced
- 1 tablespoon lemon juice
- 2 teaspoons lemon zest

Directions:
Heat up a pan with the coconut oil over medium-high heat and add the chicken, season with salt and pepper and cook for 10 minutes then transfer to a plate. Heat up the same pan over medium-high heat, add the carrots and brown them for 2-3 minutes. Top the carrots with the chicken, place in the oven and bake at 450 degrees F for 10 minutes. In a bowl, mix the couscous with the olive oil, salt, pepper, pepitas, parsley, mint, garlic, lemon juice and lemon zest. Divide the roasted chicken and carrots between plates. Add the couscous on the side and serve.
Enjoy!

Nutrition: calories 251, fat 4, fiber 6, carbs 15, protein 7

Chicken Stir Fry

Preparation time: 10 minutes
Cooking time: 10 minutes
Servings: 4

Ingredients:
- 1 ¼ pounds chicken breast, skinless, boneless and sliced
- 3 tablespoons coconut flour
- 2 tablespoons olive oil
- 1 red onion, sliced
- 2 cups sugar snap peas
- 2 garlic cloves, minced
- ½ cup teriyaki sauce
- 1 tablespoon sesame oil
- 2 tablespoons rice vinegar
- 1 tablespoon toasted sesame seeds
- 2 oranges, peeled and sliced
- 1 tablespoon chopped cilantro

Directions:
In a bowl, toss the chicken with the flour. Heat up a pan with the olive oil over medium-high heat, add the chicken, toss and cook for 4 minutes. Add the garlic and the onion, mix and cook for 1-2 minutes more. Add the sugar snap peas and cook for another 2 minutes. Add the teriyaki sauce, sesame oil, vinegar, sesame seeds, oranges and cilantro, mix and cook for 1-2 minutes. Divide everything between plates and serve.
Enjoy!

Nutrition: calories 261, fat 2, fiber 6, carbs 15, protein 6

Chicken and Veggie Soup

Preparation time: 10 minutes
Cooking time: 20 minutes
Servings: 4

Ingredients:

- 2 garlic cloves, minced
- 1 cup chopped sweet onion
- 2 zucchinis, sliced
- 2 tablespoons olive oil
- 2 teaspoons chopped dill
- 2 cups rotisserie chicken, boneless, skinless and shredded
- 7 cups chicken stock
- 1 ½ cups green beans, halved
- 5 cups baby spinach
- 2 tablespoons lemon juice

Directions:
Heat up a pot with the oil over medium-high heat, add the onion and the garlic, stir and cook for 5 minutes. Add the zucchini, dill and stock then stir and simmer for 3-4 minutes. Add the chicken and the green beans, cover the pot and simmer for 4 minutes more. Add the lemon juice, baby spinach, salt and pepper then simmer for 2 minutes, ladle into bowls and serve.
Enjoy!

Nutrition: calories 272, fat 20, fiber 6, carbs 15, protein 26

Kale and Chicken Salad

Preparation time: 10 minutes
Cooking time: 8 minutes
Servings: 4

Ingredients:

- 1½ pounds chicken tenders
- 2 teaspoons Greek seasoning
- A pinch of black pepper
- 3 tablespoons lemon juice
- 3 tablespoons olive oil
- 2 tablespoons tahini paste
- 5 ounces baby kale
- 1 garlic clove, minced
- 2 cucumbers, sliced
- 4 radishes, chopped
- 2 scallions, chopped
- 1 cup halved grape tomatoes

Directions:
Heat up a pan with half of the oil over medium-high heat, add the chicken and season with Greek seasoning and black pepper. Cook for 4 minutes on each side, transfer to a cutting board, slice and put everything in a salad bowl. Add cucumbers, kale, radishes, scallions and tomatoes and toss. In a small bowl, whisk together the rest of the oil with the lemon juice, tahini paste and garlic. Pour the dressing over the salad, toss and serve.
Enjoy!

Nutrition: calories 277, fat 4, fiber 4, carbs 14, protein 8

Chicken and Fennel Salad

Preparation time: 10 minutes
Cooking time: 8 minutes
Servings: 4

Ingredients:

- 1 ¼ pounds chicken cutlets
- 1½ teaspoon smoked paprika
- A pinch of salt and black pepper
- 3 tablespoons olive oil
- 1 fennel bulb, sliced
- ¾ cup fennel fronds
- 1/3 cup red onion, sliced
- 1 avocado, peeled, pitted and sliced
- 2 tablespoons lemon juice

Directions:

Heat up a pan with 1 tablespoon olive oil over medium-high heat then add the chicken, season with salt, pepper and smoked paprika and cook for 4 minutes on each side. Divide between plates. In a bowl, mix the rest of the oil with the fennel, fennel fronds, onion, avocado and lemon juice. Toss the salad and place next to the chicken then serve.
Enjoy!

Nutrition: calories 288, fat 4, fiber 6, carbs 12, protein 7

Shredded Chicken Salad

Preparation time: 10 minutes
Cooking time: 20 minutes
Servings: 4

Ingredients:

- 1 pound chicken breasts, skinless and boneless
- 4 parsley springs, tied
- 1 whole garlic clove+1 garlic clove, minced
- 1 bay leaf
- 1 teaspoon black peppercorns
- A pinch of salt and black pepper
- 4 cups arugula
- ½ cup chopped roasted pecans
- 1 red bell pepper, chopped
- 2 tablespoons lemon juice
- ¼ cup olive oil
- 1 teaspoon mustard
- 1 tablespoon balsamic vinegar

Directions:

Put the chicken in a pot, add water to cover and add the parsley, whole garlic clove, bay leaf, peppercorns, salt and pepper. Bring to a simmer over medium heat, cook for 20 minutes and transfer to a cutting board. Shred the chicken and put in a salad bowl. Add arugula, pecans, bell pepper, lemon juice, minced garlic, oil, mustard and vinegar then toss together and serve.
Enjoy!

Nutrition: calories 221, fat 8, fiber 5, carbs 24, protein 16

Chicken and Quinoa Pilaf

Preparation time: 10 minutes
Cooking time: 30 minutes
Servings: 4

Ingredients:

- 8 chicken thighs, skin-on and bone-in
- ¼ cup olive oil
- A pinch of salt and black pepper
- 1 cup quinoa, cooked
- 2 tablespoons rice vinegar
- 4 scallions, chopped
- 3 radishes, sliced
- 1 small carrot, grated
- ¼ cup torn basil

Directions:

Heat up a pan with half of the olive oil over medium-high heat and add the chicken. Season with salt and pepper then cook for 7 minutes and transfer the pan to the oven to roast at 450 degrees F for 20 minutes. In a bowl, mix the quinoa with the rest of the oil, salt, pepper, vinegar, scallions, radishes, carrots and basil. Divide the chicken between plates, add the quinoa pilaf on the side and serve.
Enjoy!

Nutrition: calories 213, fat 9, fiber 5, carbs 9, protein 15

Easy Roasted Chicken

Preparation time: 10 minutes
Cooking time: 1 hour and 10 minutes
Servings: 6

Ingredients:

- 2 carrots, sliced
- 3 garlic cloves, minced
- 1 yellow onion, chopped
- ½ pound sweet potatoes, cubed
- 2 tablespoons olive oil
- A pinch of salt and black pepper
- 1 thyme bunch, torn
- 1 rosemary bunch, torn
- 1 whole chicken, gizzards removed
- Juice of ½ lemon

Directions:

Put the chicken in a roasting pan and add the carrots, potatoes and onion around the chicken. Also add the oil, salt, pepper, rosemary, thyme and lemon juice to the pan. Rub the chicken a bit with the seasonings and then place the pan in the oven and bake at 425 degrees F for 1 hour and 10 minutes. Carve the chicken, divide it between plates and serve with cooking juices from the pan drizzled all over.
Enjoy!

Nutrition: calories 470, fat 17, fiber 2, carbs 12, protein 15

Grilled Chicken and Salsa

Preparation time: 30 minutes
Cooking time: 16 minutes
Servings: 4

Ingredients:

- 4 chicken breast halves, skinless and boneless
- A pinch of salt and black pepper
- ¼ cup lime juice
- 1 tablespoon lemon zest
- 4 tablespoons olive oil
- 1 teaspoon chili powder
- 1 garlic clove, minced
- 2 cups sweet cherries, pitted and chopped
- 1 small jalapeno, chopped
- 1 shallot, chopped
- ¼ cup chopped cilantro
- 1 avocado, pitted, peeled and chopped

Directions:

In a bowl, whisk the chili powder with the garlic, 3 tablespoons oil, lemon zest, salt, pepper and half of the lemon juice. Add the chicken and toss well. Cover the bowl and keep in the fridge for 30 minutes. Heat up your kitchen grill over medium-high heat, add the chicken, cook for 8 minutes on each side and divide between plates. In a separate small bowl, mix the cherries with jalapeno, shallot, cilantro, avocado, salt, pepper, the rest of the lemon juice and 1 tablespoon oil. Toss the salad well and add next to the chicken and serve.
Enjoy!

Nutrition: calories 227, fat 3, fiber 6, carbs 15, protein 9

Chicken and Broccoli

Preparation time: 10 minutes
Cooking time: 35 minutes
Servings: 4

Ingredients:

- 1 ½ tablespoons chopped rosemary
- 2 tablespoons chopped parsley
- 1 garlic clove, minced
- 2 teaspoons mustard
- 3 tablespoons olive oil
- Juice of 1 lemon
- 4 chicken breasts, skin-on and bone-in
- 1 broccoli head, florets separated
- 1 red onion, cut into wedges
- ½ teaspoon red pepper, crushed

Directions:

In a baking dish, mix the chicken with half of the oil, lemon juice, parsley, garlic, rosemary and mustard. Rub the seasonings into the chicken well then bake in the oven at 425 degrees F for 30 minutes and divide between plates once cooked. Spread the broccoli florets on a lined baking sheet, drizzle with the rest of the oil and also add the red onion and crushed pepper. Mix everything on the sheet tray together and bake in the oven at 425 degrees F for 15 minutes. Add next to the chicken and serve.
Enjoy!

Nutrition: calories 278, fat 14, fiber 6, carbs 14, protein 27

Chicken and Strawberry Salad

Preparation time: 10 minutes
Cooking time: 0 minutes
Servings: 4

Ingredients:

- 2 teaspoons lime zest
- ¼ cup olive oil
- 3 tablespoons lime juice
- 1½ tablespoon raw honey
- A pinch of salt and black pepper
- 1 romaine lettuce head, torn
- 2 cups halved strawberries
- 2 chicken breasts, grilled and sliced
- 1 cup canned peas, drained and rinsed
- ½ cup sliced red onion
- 1 avocado, pitted, peeled and cubed

Directions:

In a bowl, mix the chicken with lime zest, lime juice, salt, pepper, lettuce, strawberries, peas, onion and avocado. Add the oil and the honey, toss and serve.
Enjoy!

Nutrition: calories 271, fat 4, fiber 8, carbs 16, protein 8

Greek Chicken Mix

Preparation time: 10 minutes
Cooking time: 30 minutes
Servings: 4

Ingredients:

- 1 tablespoon lemon zest
- 2 tablespoons lemon juice
- 1 tablespoon chopped thyme
- 1 ½ teaspoons Greek seasoning
- 5 tablespoons olive oil
- 3 garlic cloves, minced
- 4 chicken breasts, skinless and boneless
- 1 cup rice, cooked
- ¼ cup veggie stock
- 1 cup grape tomatoes, halved
- 3 small cucumbers, sliced
- 3 scallions, chopped
- 1 cup chopped parsley
- ¼ cup chopped mint

Directions:

In a baking dish, mix the chicken with the lemon zest, half of the lemon juice, thyme, garlic, Greek seasoning, stock and 2 tablespoons oil. Rub the seasonings into the chicken well then bake in the oven at 400 degrees F for 30 minutes. Once cooked, divide between plates. In a bowl, mix the rice with the rest of the lemon juice, tomatoes, cucumbers, scallions, parsley, mint, salt and pepper then toss and add next to the chicken and serve.
Enjoy!

Nutrition: calories 288, fat 6, fiber 5, carbs 14, protein 20

Spring Chicken Mix

Preparation time: 10 minutes
Cooking time: 20 minutes
Servings: 4

Ingredients:

- 4 chicken breasts, skinless and boneless
- A pinch of salt and black pepper
- 3 tablespoons coconut oil
- 1 shallot, chopped
- 1 cup vegetable stock
- 1½ cups snow peas
- 1½ cups sugar snap peas
- 1½ cups sliced asparagus
- 2 teaspoons lemon zest
- 2 garlic cloves, minced
- 1 tablespoon chopped tarragon

Directions:

Heat up a pan with 1 tablespoon oil over medium-high heat and add the chicken, season with salt and pepper, cook for 6-7 minutes on each side and transfer to a plate once cooked. Heat up the same pan over medium-high heat, add the shallot, stir and cook for 1 minute. Add the stock, the rest of the oil, snow peas, lemon zest, sugar snap peas, asparagus, garlic and tarragon to the pan. Stir and cook for 4-5 minutes more. Divide the chicken between plates and serve with the veggie mix on the side.
Enjoy!

Nutrition: calories 271, fat 6, fiber 7, carbs 8, protein 16

Delicious Chicken Drumsticks Mix

Preparation time: 10 minutes
Cooking time: 50 minutes
Servings: 4

Ingredients:

- 2 tablespoons olive oil
- 8 chicken drumsticks
- A pinch of salt and black pepper
- ¾ cup chicken stock
- ½ cup coconut cream
- 1 red onion, cut into wedges
- Juice of ¼ lemon
- 3 garlic cloves, minced
- 1 pound carrots, sliced
- 1 pound baby red potatoes, halved
- 1 tablespoon mustard
- 1 ½ tablespoons chopped tarragon

Directions:

Put the chicken drumsticks in a baking dish, add the olive oil, salt, pepper, onion, garlic, stock, carrots and potatoes then toss everything together. In a bowl, whisk the cream with lemon juice, mustard and tarragon and pour over the chicken. Toss everything again and place in the oven at 450 degrees F, bake for 50 minutes, divide between plates and serve.
Enjoy!

Nutrition: calories 265, fat 8, fiber 7, carbs 16, protein 20

Chicken and Dill Soup

Preparation time: 10 minutes
Cooking time: 45 minutes
Servings: 8

Ingredients:

- 3 carrots, sliced
- 2 tablespoons olive oil
- 3 celery stalks, chopped
- 3 garlic cloves, minced
- 1 small onion, chopped
- 3 chicken breasts, skinless and boneless
- 8 cups chicken stock
- 2 bay leaves
- 3 thyme springs
- A pinch of salt and black pepper
- 4 cups baby spinach
- 3 tablespoons chopped dill
- 1 tablespoons lemon zest
- 2 tablespoons lemon juice

Directions:

Heat up a pot with the oil over medium-high heat, add the celery, carrots, onion and garlic, stir and cook for 5 minutes. Add the chicken, stock, bay leaves, thyme, salt and pepper. Stir, bring to a boil, cover, reduce heat and simmer for 20 minutes. Discard thyme and bay leaves then transfer the chicken to a cutting board and shred it. Return it to the pot and cook everything for 10 minutes more. Add dill, spinach, lemon juice and lemon zest. Mix well and ladle into bowls and serve.
Enjoy!
Nutrition: calories 229, fat 5, fiber 9, carbs 15, protein 18

Chicken Minestrone

Preparation time: 10 minutes
Cooking time: 8 hours
Servings: 4

Ingredients:

- 1 yellow onion, chopped
- 1 fennel bulb, chopped
- 2 carrots, sliced
- 2 garlic cloves, minced
- 6 cups chicken stock
- 28 ounces canned tomatoes, chopped
- 15 ounces canned kidney beans, drained and rinsed
- 2 teaspoons dried oregano
- 2 teaspoons dried basil
- A pinch of salt and black pepper
- 1 bay leaf
- 4 chicken thighs, bone-in and skinless
- ½ bunch kale, chopped
- 2/3 cup quinoa
- 6 ounces green beans, halved

Directions:

In a slow cooker, combine the onion with fennel, carrots, garlic, stock, tomatoes, beans, oregano, basil, salt, pepper, bay leaf and chicken. Toss, cover and cook on Low for 7 hours and 30 minutes. Add the kale, quinoa and green beans, cover the pot again and cook on Low for 30 minutes more. Divide into bowls and serve.
Enjoy!
Nutrition: calories 299, fat 3, fiber 7, carbs 23, protein 19

Chicken Thigh and Salsa Verde

Preparation time: 10 minutes
Cooking time: 25 minutes
Servings: 4

Ingredients:

- 1¼ cups chicken stock
- 2 teaspoons olive oil
- 6 chicken thighs, bone-in and skin-on
- A pinch of salt and black pepper
- 3 red bell peppers, chopped
- ½ yellow onion, chopped
- 2 garlic cloves
- 1 cup couscous, cooked

For the Salsa Verde:

- ¼ cup chopped basil
- ¼ cup chopped parsley
- 1 green onion, chopped
- ¼ cup olive oil
- 2 tablespoons capers
- 1½ tablespoons lemon juice

Directions:

Put the stock in a pot, bring to a boil over medium heat, add the couscous, cover and leave aside for 10 minutes. Fluff the couscous with a fork and set it aside for now. Heat up a pan with the oil over medium-high heat, add the chicken, season with salt and pepper, cook for 10 minutes skin side down, flip, cook for 4 minutes more and transfer to a plate. Heat up the same pan over medium heat, add the onion, garlic, and bell peppers, stir and cook for 2-3 minutes more. Add the chicken, toss and divide between plates. Add the couscous on the side and leave aside for now. In a bowl, mix the basil with parsley, green onion, capers, lemon juice and oil and stir well. Drizzle this over the chicken and couscous mix and serve.
Enjoy!

Nutrition: calories 300, fat 15, fiber 7, carbs 11, protein 16

Chicken and Beets

Preparation time: 10 minutes
Cooking time: 8 hours
Servings: 5

Ingredients:

- 1 whole chicken, cut into medium pieces
- A pinch of salt and black pepper
- 2 teaspoons sweet paprika
- 1 ½ teaspoon thyme, dried
- Juice of 1 lemon
- 1 red onion, cut into wedges
- 1 celery rib, chopped
- ½ pound baby carrots
- 4 garlic cloves, minced
- 1 pounds assorted beets, peeled and quartered
- 12 Brussels sprouts
- 1½ teaspoon mustard
- 1 tablespoon chopped rosemary

Directions:

In your slow cooker, mix the onion with celery, carrots, garlic, sprouts, beets, mustard and rosemary. Add chicken pieces, paprika, thyme, salt, pepper and lemon juice. Toss everything, cover, cook on Low for 8 hours then divide into bowls and serve.
Enjoy!
Nutrition: calories 297, fat 7, fiber 6, carbs 11, protein 19

Indian Chicken Salad

Preparation time: 10 minutes
Cooking time: 0 minutes
Servings: 4

Ingredients:

- 1 cup coconut cream
- 2 teaspoons curry powder
- ½ cup grapes
- A pinch of salt and black pepper
- ¼ cup chopped walnuts
- 1 lettuce head, torn
- 2 cups chicken, cooked and shredded

Directions:

In a bowl, mix the chicken with the lettuce, walnuts, salt, pepper, grapes, curry powder and cream, toss and serve right away.
Enjoy!

Nutrition: calories 222, fat 9, fiber 7, carbs 14, protein 17

Chicken and Berries Salad

Preparation time: 10 minutes
Cooking time: 14 minutes
Servings: 4

Ingredients:

- ¼ cup balsamic vinegar
- ½ cup olive oil
- 2 tablespoons orange juice
- A pinch of salt and black pepper
- Cooking spray
- 1 pound chicken breasts, skinless and boneless
- ½ cup raspberries
- ½ cup blueberries
- ½ cup pecans, roasted
- 8 ounces sugar snap peas
- 1 cup sliced strawberries
- 8 cups mixed salad greens

Directions:

Heat up a grill over medium-high heat then add the chicken, spray with cooking oil, season with a pinch of salt and black pepper. Cook for 7 minutes on each side then transfer to a cutting board, cut into thin strips and put in a salad bowl. Add raspberries, blueberries, pecans, snap peas, strawberries, salad greens, orange juice, oil and vinegar, toss and serve.
Enjoy!

Nutrition: calories 300, fat 12, fiber 7, carbs 15, protein 18

Tarragon Chicken Salad

Preparation time: 10 minutes
Cooking time: 0 minutes
Servings: 4

Ingredients:

- 1/3 cup coconut cream
- ¼ cup canola mayonnaise
- 1 tablespoon chopped tarragon, chopped
- A pinch of salt and black pepper
- 2 cups rotisserie chicken, skinless, boneless and shredded
- ¼ cup sliced red onion

Directions:
In a salad bowl, mix the chicken with onion, salt, pepper, tarragon, mayo and cream then serve.
Enjoy!

Nutrition: calories 298, fat 8, fiber 4, carbs 14, protein 15

Chicken and Mushrooms Soup

Preparation time: 10 minutes
Cooking time: 15 minutes
Servings: 4

Ingredients:

- 2 tablespoons olive oil
- 3 garlic cloves, minced
- 8 ounces baby Bella mushrooms, sliced
- 3 carrots, sliced
- 1 yellow onion, chopped
- 2 celery stalks, chopped
- ¼ cup coconut cream
- 1 tablespoon chopped thyme
- 4 cups chicken stock
- 1 cup coconut milk
- 1 cup brown rice
- 2 chicken breasts, skinless, boneless and cubed

Directions:
Heat up a pot with the oil over medium heat then add carrots, mushrooms, onion and celery, stir and cook for 6 minutes. Add the chicken, toss and cook for 5 minutes more. Add thyme, garlic, salt, pepper, stock and milk. Stir well and cook for 2-3 minutes. Add the rice, stir, bring to a simmer over medium heat and cook for 10 more minutes until the rice is done. Divide the soup into bowls and serve.
Enjoy!

Nutrition: calories 300, fat 6, fiber 7, carbs 15, protein 16

Chicken and Plum Sauce

Preparation time: 10 minutes
Cooking time: 1 hour and 40 minutes
Servings: 6

Ingredients:
- 1 whole chicken
- A pinch of salt and black pepper
- 1 red onion, chopped
- 3 tablespoons olive oil
- 1 teaspoon grated fresh ginger
- 4 garlic cloves, minced
- 21-ounces plums, stones removed and chopped
- 6 tablespoons coconut aminos
- 1 tablespoon balsamic vinegar
- 4 tablespoons sriracha

Directions:
Arrange the chicken in a roasting pan and season with salt and pepper. Drizzle half of the oil over the chicken and rub the seasonings and oil into the chicken. Place in the oven at 400 degrees F and roast for 1 hour and 10 minutes. Heat up a pan with the rest of the oil over medium heat then add onion, stir and cook for 5 minutes. Add the garlic, ginger, plums, coconut aminos, sriracha and vinegar. Stir, bring to a simmer and cook for 20 minutes. Transfer this mix to your blender, pulse a few times and then brush the cooked chicken with this mix. Cook the chicken for 10 minutes more in the oven then carve and serve with the sauce from the pan drizzled all over. Enjoy!

Nutrition: calories 280, fat 8, fiber 4, carbs 12, protein 17

Adobo Chicken Mix

Preparation time: 10 minutes
Cooking time: 40 minutes
Servings: 6

Ingredients:
- 6 chicken thighs
- Salt and black pepper to the taste
- 1 tablespoon olive oil
- Zest of 1 lime
- 1½ teaspoons chipotle peppers in adobo sauce
- 1 cup sliced peach
- 1 tablespoon lime juice

Directions:
Heat up a pan with the oil over medium-high heat and add the chicken thighs. Season with salt and pepper then brown for 4 minutes on each side and bake in the oven at 375 degrees F for 20 minutes. In your food processor, mix the peaches with the chipotle, lime zest and lime juice then blend and pour over the chicken. Bake for 10 minutes more, divide everything between plates and serve.
Enjoy!

Nutrition: calories 309, fat 6, fiber 4, carbs 16, protein 15

Chicken and Rice

Preparation time: 10 minutes
Cooking time: 25 minutes
Servings: 2

Ingredients:
- 2 tablespoons coconut oil
- 8 ounces chicken breast, cubed
- 3 tablespoons almond flour
- Salt and black pepper to the taste

For the cauliflower rice:
- 3 cups chopped cauliflower
- 2 tablespoons coconut flakes
- 2 teaspoons coconut oil
- 1 mango, cored and cubed
- 1 tablespoon chopped cilantro
- 1 tablespoon chopped green onions
- 1 tablespoon sesame seeds, toasted

Directions:
In a bowl, mix the almond flour with the chicken, salt and pepper and toss to coat. Heat up a pan with 2 tablespoons coconut oil over medium-high heat then add chicken, stir, cook for 5 minutes on each side and divide between plates. In your food processor, mix cauliflower with salt and pepper and blend well to turn the cauliflower into "rice". Heat up a pan with 2 teaspoons coconut oil over medium-high heat. Add cauliflower and coconut flakes, stir and cook for 3 minutes. Reduce heat and add mango, cilantro, green onions and sesame seeds. Stir, cover the pan, cook for 5 minutes more. Divide between two plates and serve next to the chicken. Enjoy!

Nutrition: calories 260, fat 22, fiber 6, carbs 13, protein 19

Chicken and Raspberry Sauce

Preparation time: 10 minutes
Cooking time: 25 minutes
Servings: 2

Ingredients:
- 1 shallot, chopped
- 2 chicken breasts, skinless and boneless
- 2 garlic cloves, minced
- 1/3 cup balsamic vinegar
- 1 cup chicken stock
- 2 tablespoons coconut oil
- 2 cups raspberries
- Salt and black pepper to the taste

Directions:
Heat up a pan with half of the coconut oil over medium-high heat. Add the chicken, season with salt and pepper and cook for 5 minutes. Place the chicken in the oven, roast for 10 minutes at 325 degrees F then divide between plates. Meanwhile, heat up the pan with the rest of the oil over medium-high heat and add shallot and garlic, stir and cook for 3 minutes. Add vinegar, stock, raspberries, salt and pepper. Stir, cook for 5 minutes more, drizzle over the chicken and serve. Enjoy!

Nutrition: calories 280, fat 6, fiber 3, carbs 15, protein 16

Slow Cooked Chicken Curry

Preparation time: 10 minutes
Cooking time: 5 hours
Servings: 4

Ingredients:

- 2 sweet potatoes, cubed
- 3 chicken breasts, boneless, skinless and chopped
- 1 red bell pepper, chopped
- 1 small yellow onion, chopped
- 2 cups coconut milk
- 2 cups chicken stock
- 1 teaspoon ground cumin
- 3 tablespoons curry powder
- 2 tablespoons chopped cilantro
- Salt and cayenne pepper to the taste

Directions:

In your slow cooker, mix the chicken the sweet potatoes, bell pepper, onion, stock, milk, cumin, curry powder, salt and cayenne. Cover and cook on Low for 5 hours then divide into bowls, sprinkle the cilantro on top and serve.
Enjoy!

Nutrition: calories 280, fat 13, fiber 7, carbs 8, protein 15

Cumin Chicken Mix

Preparation time: 2 hours
Cooking time: 25 minutes
Servings: 4

Ingredients:

- 4 garlic cloves, minced
- 2 pounds chicken thighs, skinless and boneless
- 4 tablespoons extra-virgin olive oil
- 4 tablespoons chopped cilantro
- 2 tablespoons lime juice
- A pinch of salt and black pepper
- 2 tablespoons olive oil
- 1 teaspoon cumin, ground
- 1 teaspoon red chili flakes
- Lime wedges for serving

Directions:

In a bowl, whisk the olive oil with salt, pepper, cilantro, garlic, lime juice, cumin and chili flakes. Add the chicken, toss, cover and leave aside for 2 hours. Heat up a pan with the oil over medium-high heat, add chicken, cook for 3 minutes on each side and transfer to a baking dish. Cook in the oven at 375 degrees F for 20 minutes then divide between plates and serve with lime wedges on the side.
Enjoy!

Nutrition: calories 200, fat 10, fiber 1, carbs 12, protein 24

Rosemary Chicken Thighs

Preparation time: 10 minutes
Cooking time: 40 minutes
Servings: 2

Ingredients:

- 14 ounces chicken thighs, bone-in
- 1 tablespoon lemon juice
- 1 teaspoon chili powder
- A pinch of salt and black pepper
- 1 tablespoon fresh minced ginger
- 1 tablespoon olive oil
- 4 onions, chopped
- 2 rosemary springs, chopped

Directions:

In a bowl, mix chili powder with lemon juice and ginger. Add the chicken, rub it with this mix and then let sit for 10 minutes. Heat up a pan with the oil over medium-high heat, add the marinated chicken pieces and cook for 3 minutes on each side. Add rosemary, onions, salt and pepper. Reduce heat to medium, cover pan, cook for 25 minutes. Divide between plates and serve.
Enjoy!

Nutrition: calories 210, fat 8, fiber 9, carbs 12, protein 17

Turkey Stew

Preparation time: 10 minutes
Cooking time: 1 hour and 20 minutes
Servings: 6

Ingredients:

- 3 teaspoons olive oil
- 1 green bell pepper, chopped
- 1 pound ground turkey meat
- 1 tablespoons garlic, minced
- 1 yellow onion, chopped
- 1 teaspoon ground ancho chilies
- 1 tablespoon chili powder
- 2 teaspoons ground cumin
- 8 ounces canned green chilies and juice, chopped
- 8 ounces tomato paste
- 15 ounces canned tomatoes, chopped
- 2 cups veggie stock
- A pinch of salt and black pepper

Directions:

Heat up a pan with 2 teaspoons oil over medium heat, add turkey, stir, brown well on all sides and transfer to a pot. Heat up the pan with the rest of the oil over medium heat and add onion and green bell pepper. Stir and cook for 3 minutes. Add garlic, chili powder, ancho chili powder, salt, pepper and cumin, stir and cook for 2 more minutes. Transfer this to the pot with the turkey meat, add chilies and juice, tomato sauce, chopped tomatoes, stock, salt and pepper. Stir, bring to a boil, cover the pot and cook for 1 hour. Divide into bowls and serve.
Enjoy!

Nutrition: calories 327, fat 8, fiber 13, carbs 24, protein 27

Chicken and Mushroom Salad

Preparation time: 10 minutes
Cooking time: 0 minutes
Servings: 4

Ingredients:

- 1 yellow onion, chopped
- 12 ounces canned mushrooms, drained and chopped
- 2 garlic cloves, minced
- 2 teaspoons chopped rosemary
- 3 cups chicken, already cooked and shredded
- 2 cups baby spinach
- Salt and black pepper to the tastes
- A splash of balsamic vinegar
- A drizzle of olive oil

Directions:

In a bowl, mix the mushrooms with the chicken, onion, garlic, rosemary, spinach, salt, pepper, vinegar and oil, toss and serve.
Enjoy!

Nutrition: calories 210, fat 5, fiber 8, carbs 15, protein 11

Chicken Roast

Preparation time: 10 minutes
Cooking time: 1 hour and 10 minutes
Servings: 4

Ingredients:

- 1 whole chicken
- A pinch of salt and black pepper
- 2 tablespoons olive oil
- 2 green onions, chopped
- 1 cup chicken stock
- 2 teaspoons lemon juice
- 2 teaspoons chopped rosemary

Directions:

Place chicken in a roasting pan, add salt, pepper, oil, green onions, stock, lemon juice and rosemary. Toss the ingredients together, place in the oven and bake at 450 degrees F for 1 hour. Slice the meat, divide it between plates and serve with cooking juices drizzled on top.
Enjoy!

Nutrition: calories 495, fat 8, fiber 4, carbs 10, protein 27

Ginger Chicken Thighs

Preparation time: 12 hours
Cooking time: 1 hour
Servings: 4

Ingredients:
- 8 chicken thighs, bone in and skin on
- A pinch of sea salt and black pepper
- 1 tablespoon apple cider vinegar
- 3 tablespoons chopped onion
- 1 tablespoon fresh grated ginger
- ½ teaspoon dried thyme
- ¾ cup apple juice
- ½ cup maple syrup

Directions:
In a bowl, combine chicken thighs with salt, pepper, vinegar, onion, ginger, thyme, apple juice and maple syrup. Cover and keep in the fridge for 12 hours to marinate. Transfer this whole mix to a baking dish, cover dish, bake in the oven at 400 degrees F for 1 hour. Divide the meat and sauce between plates and serve.
Enjoy!

Nutrition: calories 274, fat 6, fiber 8, carbs 14, protein 12

Thai Chicken Thighs

Preparation time: 10 minutes
Cooking time: 6 hours and 10 minutes
Servings: 6

Ingredients:
- 4 pounds chicken thighs, skin-on and bone-in
- 1 bunch green onions, chopped
- ½ cup Thai sweet chili sauce

Directions:
Heat up a pan over medium-high heat, add chicken thighs and brown them for 5 minutes on each side. Transfer the chicken to your slow cooker, add green onions and chili sauce, cover and cook on Low for 6 hours. Divide between plates and serve.
Enjoy!

Nutrition: calories 260, fat 4, fiber 2, carbs 12, protein 14

Chicken with Parsley Sauce

Preparation time: 30 minutes
Cooking time: 40 minutes
Servings: 6
Ingredients:

- 1 cup chopped parsley
- 1 teaspoon dried oregano
- ½ cup olive oil
- ¼ cup vegetable stock
- 4 garlic cloves
- A pinch of salt and black pepper
- 12 chicken thighs

Directions:

In your food processor, mix parsley with oregano, garlic, salt, oil and the stock. Pulse well until smooth. In a bowl, mix the chicken with the parsley sauce and toss, cover and keep in the fridge for 30 minutes. Heat up your kitchen grill over medium heat and place the chicken pieces on the grill. Close the lid and cook for 20 minutes. Flip the chicken and cook for 20 minutes more. Divide between plates and serve with the parsley sauce on top.
Enjoy!

Nutrition: calories 254, fat 3, fiber 3, carbs 7, protein 12

Chicken and Lentil Casserole

Preparation time: 10 minutes
Cooking time: 1 hour and 40 minutes
Servings: 8
Ingredients:

- 1½ cups green lentils
- 3 cups clean chicken stock
- 2 pound chicken breasts, skinless, boneless and cubed
- A pinch of sea salt and cayenne pepper
- 3 teaspoons ground cumin
- Cooking spray
- 5 garlic cloves, minced
- 1 yellow onion, chopped
- 2 red bell peppers, chopped
- 14 ounces canned tomatoes, chopped
- 2 cups corn
- 2 tablespoons chopped jalapeno pepper
- 1 tablespoon garlic powder
- 1 cup chopped parsley

Directions:

Put the stock in a pot, add a pinch of salt and the lentils. Stir, bring to a boil over medium heat, cover and simmer for 35 minutes. Heat up a pan with some cooking spray over medium-high heat and add the chicken, season with salt, cayenne pepper and 1 teaspoon cumin. Cook for 5 minutes on each side then transfer to a bowl. Heat up the pan again over medium heat, add bell peppers, garlic, onion, tomatoes, salt, cayenne and 1 teaspoon cumin. Stir, cook for 7 minutes and transfer to the bowl with the chicken. Drain the lentils, add them to the bowl with the meat and then add jalapeno pepper, garlic powder, the rest of the cumin, corn and parsley. Toss, transfer the whole mix to a baking dish and place in the oven at 350 degrees F and bake for 50 minutes. Divide between plates and serve.
Enjoy!

Nutrition: calories 244, fat 11, fiber 4, carbs 10, protein 13

Chicken Breasts and Mushrooms

Preparation time: 10 minutes
Cooking time: 30 minutes
Servings: 6

Ingredients:

- 3 pounds chicken breasts, skinless and boneless
- 1 yellow onion, chopped
- 1 garlic clove, minced
- A pinch of salt and black pepper
- 10 mushrooms, chopped
- 1 tablespoon olive oil
- 2 red bell peppers, chopped

Directions:

Put chicken in a baking dish, add onion, garlic, salt, pepper, mushrooms, oil and bell peppers. Mix briefly and bake in the oven at 425 degrees F for 30 minutes. Divide between plates and serve.
Enjoy!

Nutrition: calories 285, fat 12, fiber 1, carbs 13, protein 16

Asian Chicken and Cauliflower

Preparation time: 10 minutes
Cooking time: 25 minutes
Servings: 4

Ingredients:

- 2 pounds chicken breasts, skinless, boneless and cubed
- 1 tablespoon rice vinegar
- 4 tablespoons raw honey
- 6 tablespoons coconut aminos
- 2 garlic cloves, minced
- 2 pounds cauliflower, florets separated
- ½ cup water
- 1 tablespoon whole wheat flour
- 2 tablespoons olive oil
- 3 green onions, chopped
- 2 tablespoons sesame seeds

Directions:

In a bowl, mix 3 tablespoons honey with 3 tablespoons coconut aminos, garlic, vinegar and the chicken. Heat up a pan with half of the oil over medium heat, add cauliflower and stir then cook for 5 minutes and transfer to a bowl. Heat up the pan with the rest of the oil over medium heat, Drain the chicken, reserving the marinade, then add it to the pan. Toss and cook for 6 minutes. In a separate bowl, whisk together the rest of the aminos with the remaining honey, water, whole wheat flour and the reserved marinade. Add over the chicken, cover the pan and cook on low heat for 10 minutes, take off the heat, add the cauliflower and toss. Divide between plates, sprinkle green onions and sesame seeds on top and serve.
Enjoy!

Nutrition: calories 250, fat 4, fiber 5, carbs 10, protein 12

Chicken and Corn Soup

Preparation time: 10 minutes
Cooking time: 8 hours
Servings: 6

Ingredients:
- 8 cups chicken stock
- 2 teaspoons garlic powder
- A pinch of salt and black pepper
- 14 ounces coconut milk
- 1½ cups green lentils
- 2 pounds chicken breasts, skinless, boneless and cubed
- 1/3 cup chopped parsley
- 3 cups corn
- 3 handfuls spinach
- 3 green onions, chopped

Directions:
In your slow cooker, mix the stock with salt, pepper, chicken, lentils, garlic powder and corn. Cover and cook on Low for 7 hours and 30 minutes. Add the coconut milk, spinach and green onions the recover and cook on Low for 30 minutes more. Add the parsley, stir, divide into bowls and serve.
Enjoy!

Nutrition: calories 265, fat 8, fiber 10, carbs 10, protein 24

Chicken and Artichoke Stew

Preparation time: 10 minutes
Cooking time: 1 hour
Servings: 8

Ingredients:
- 2 yellow onions, chopped
- 2 pounds chicken thighs, skinless, boneless and chopped
- 5 garlic cloves, minced
- 2 tablespoons olive oil
- 16 ounces canned artichoke hearts, drained and chopped
- 1 tablespoon maple syrup
- 2 cups vegetable stock
- A pinch of sea salt and black pepper
- 2 tablespoons chopped cilantro

Directions:
Heat up a pot with half of the oil over medium heat, add chicken, cook for 4 minutes on each side and transfer to a bowl. Heat up the pot again with the rest of the oil over medium-high heat, add garlic and onion then stir and cook for 1 minute. Add the stock, maple syrup, artichokes, salt and pepper. Stir well, bring to a simmer and cook for 3-4 minutes. Return chicken to the pot, stir, cover, reduce heat to low and cook for 45 minutes. Add the cilantro, toss, divide into bowls and serve.
Enjoy!

Nutrition: calories 200, fat 4, fiber 4, carbs 10, protein 16

Chicken Bites and Green Beans

Preparation time: 10 minutes
Cooking time: 30 minutes
Servings: 4

Ingredients:
- 1½ pounds chicken breasts, cubed
- 2 tablespoons olive oil
- 2 pounds green beans, trimmed
- 25 ounces canned tomato sauce
- 2 tablespoons chopped parsley
- 6 ounces canned tomato paste
- A pinch of salt and black pepper

Directions:
Heat up a pan with half of the oil over medium heat, add chicken, stir, cook for 5 minutes on each side and transfer to a bowl. Set the cooked chicken aside. Heat up the pan with the rest of the oil over medium heat, add green beans, stir and cook for 10 minutes. Return chicken to the pan, add salt, pepper, tomato sauce, tomato paste and parsley. Stir and cook for 5 minutes more then divide between plates and serve.
Enjoy!

Nutrition: calories 250, fat 4, fiber 2, carbs 6, protein 12

Pumpkin and Chicken Soup

Preparation time: 10 minutes
Cooking time: 20 minutes
Servings: 4

Ingredients:
- 2 chicken breasts, skinless, boneless and cubed
- 1 yellow onion, chopped
- 2 tablespoons olive oil
- 1 garlic clove, chopped
- 20 ounces pumpkin , peeled, seedless and cubed
- 2 carrots, chopped
- ½ teaspoon fresh grated ginger
- ½ teaspoon ground cumin
- 1 teaspoon ground turmeric
- A pinch of salt and black pepper
- 12 ounces coconut milk
- 16 ounces chicken stock

Directions:
Heat up a pot with the oil over medium-high heat then add garlic and onion. Stir and cook for 2 minutes. Add carrots, pumpkin, ginger, cumin, turmeric, stock, coconut milk and chicken, Stir, bring to a boil, reduce heat to medium and simmer for 15 minutes. Add salt and pepper, blend slightly using an immersion blender then divide into bowls and serve.
Enjoy!

Nutrition: calories 220, fat 3, fiber 9, carbs 7, protein 11

Kale and Chicken Soup

Preparation time: 10 minutes
Cooking time: 15 minutes
Servings: 2

Ingredients:

- 1 red bell pepper, chopped
- 1 yellow onion, chopped
- ¼ cup chopped pickled jalapeno peppers
- 2 garlic cloves, minced
- 1 tablespoon olive oil
- 1 teaspoon ground cumin
- 1 teaspoon ground coriander
- 1 teaspoon dried oregano
- 1 ½ cups chicken breast, cooked and shredded
- 2 ½ cups chicken stock
- 2 cups kale, torn
- Zest of 1 lime, grated
- Juice of 1 lime
- A pinch of salt and black pepper
- 15 ounces canned tomatoes, chopped
- 2 tablespoons chopped spring onions
- 1 avocado, peeled, pitted and sliced
- 1 teaspoon sweet paprika
- 3 tablespoons chopped coriander

Directions:

Heat up a pot with the oil over medium heat, add onion, stir and cook for 2 minutes. Add red bell peppers, garlic, jalapenos, oregano, cumin, coriander, tomatoes, kale, chicken, lime zest, stock, lime juice, salt and pepper. Stir the mix, bring to a boil, cook for 10 minutes and take off heat. Ladle soup into bowls, top with green onion, paprika, chopped coriander and avocado and serve. Enjoy!

Nutrition: calories 170, fat 3, fiber 3, carbs 12, protein 11

Chicken and Sweet Potatoes Stew

Preparation time: 10 minutes
Cooking time: 8 hours
Servings: 4

Ingredients:

- 2 carrots, chopped
- 5 garlic cloves, minced
- 2 celery sticks, chopped
- 2 onions, chopped
- 2 sweet potatoes, cubed
- 14 ounces tomato juice
- 1-quart chicken stock
- 2 cups chicken meat, skinless, boneless and cubed
- A pinch of salt and black pepper
- ¼ teaspoon cayenne pepper
- ½ pound baby spinach

Directions:

In your slow cooker, combine the carrots with the garlic, celery, onions, sweet potatoes, tomato juice, stock, chicken, salt, pepper and cayenne. Mix and cover then cook on Low for 7 hours and 40 minutes. Add the spinach, cover and cook on Low for 20 minutes more. Divide into bowls and serve.
Enjoy!

Nutrition: calories 250, fat 3, fiber 3, carbs 14, protein 7

Chicken and Carrot Stew

Preparation time: 10 minutes
Cooking time: 7 hours
Servings: 4

Ingredients:

- 2 tablespoons olive oil
- 8 carrots, chopped
- 1 ½ pounds chicken breasts, skinless, boneless and cubed
- ½ teaspoon black peppercorns
- 1 yellow onion, chopped
- ¼ cup tapioca flour
- 1 tablespoon chopped thyme
- 4 cups chicken stock
- A pinch of salt and black pepper

Directions:
Heat up a pan with the oil over medium-high heat, add the chicken and stir. Brown for 4 minutes on all sides and transfer to your slow cooker. Add the carrots, peppercorns, onion, tapioca, thyme, stock, salt and pepper to the slow cooker as well. Stir, cover and cook on Low for 7 hours. Divide into bowls and serve.
Enjoy!

Nutrition: calories 260, fat 8, fiber 5, carbs 14, protein 11

Turkey and Squash Soup

Preparation time: 10 minutes
Cooking time: 35 minutes
Servings: 4

Ingredients:

- 3 celery stalks, chopped
- 1 yellow onion, chopped
- 1 tablespoon olive oil
- 6 cups chicken stock
- Salt and black pepper to the taste
- ¼ cup chopped parsley
- 3 cups baked spaghetti squash, chopped
- 3 cups turkey, cooked and shredded

Directions:
Heat up a pot with the oil over medium-high heat, add celery and onion then stir and cook for 5 minutes. Add parsley, stock, turkey meat, salt and pepper. Stir and cook for 20 minutes. Add spaghetti squash, stir, cook for 10 minutes more, divide into bowls and serve.
Enjoy!

Nutrition: calories 180, fat 4, fiber 8, carbs 11, protein 10

Turkey Casserole

Preparation time: 10 minutes
Cooking time: 45 minutes
Servings: 8

Ingredients:
- 4 cups spiralized zucchinis
- 1 egg, whisked
- 3 cups shredded cabbage
- 3 cups turkey meat, cooked and shredded
- ½ cup chicken stock
- ½ cup coconut cream
- Salt and black pepper to the taste
- ¼ teaspoon garlic powder

Directions:
Heat up a pan with the stock over medium-low heat, add the egg, cream, salt, pepper and garlic powder. Stir and bring to a simmer then add the cabbage and the turkey. Stir and take off the heat. Arrange the zucchini noodles in a baking dish and pour turkey mix on top as well. Spread the mix across the pan then cover the dish and bake in the oven at 400 degrees F for 35 minutes. Divide between plates and serve.
Enjoy!

Nutrition: calories 240, fat 15, fiber 1, carbs 9, protein 15

Coconut Chicken Dish

Preparation time: 10 minutes
Cooking time: 50 minutes
Servings: 4

Ingredients:
- 3 pounds chicken breasts, boneless and skinless
- Cooking spray
- 4 ounces coconut cream
- 1 zucchini, shredded
- 1 carrot, shredded
- Salt and black pepper to the taste
- 1 teaspoon minced garlic

Directions:
In a bowl, mix the cream with the zucchini, carrot, garlic, salt and pepper. Arrange the chicken in a baking dish greased with cooking spray then add the cream mixture and spread evenly into the pan. Place in the oven at 400 degrees F, bake for 45 minutes, divide between plates and serve.
Enjoy!

Nutrition: calories 425, fat 5, fiber 1, carbs 8, protein 20

Chicken and Veggies

Preparation time: 10 minutes
Cooking time: 40 minutes
Servings: 6

Ingredients:
- 2 cups coconut cream
- 40 ounces rotisserie chicken pieces, boneless, skinless and shredded
- 3 tablespoons coconut oil, melted
- ½ cup chopped yellow onion
- ¾ cup chopped red peppers
- 29 ounces chicken stock
- Salt and black pepper to the taste
- 8 ounces mushrooms, chopped
- 1 cup green beans
- 17 ounces asparagus, trimmed
- 3 teaspoons chopped thyme

Directions:
Heat up a pan with the cream over medium heat, bring to a simmer and cook for 6-7 minutes. Heat up a pan with the oil over medium heat, add onion and peppers, stir and cook for 3 minutes. Add stock, salt and pepper and then bring to a boil and cook for 10 minutes. Add asparagus, green beans and mushrooms, stir and cook for 7 minutes. Add chicken pieces, cream, thyme, salt and pepper. Stir and cook for 3-4 minutes more then divide between plates and serve. Enjoy!

Nutrition: calories 430, fat 27, fiber 3, carbs 4, protein 47

Avocado and Chicken Salad

Preparation time: 10 minutes
Cooking time: 0 minutes
Servings: 2

Ingredients:
- 1 avocado, pitted, peeled and sliced
- Salt and black pepper to the taste
- 3 tablespoons coconut cream
- 1 chicken breast, grilled and shredded

Directions:
In a salad bowl, mix the avocado with the chicken, salt, pepper and coconut cream. Toss well and serve right away
Enjoy!

Nutrition: calories 218, fat 14, fiber 5, carbs 10, protein 15

Egg and Chicken Salad

Preparation time: 10 minutes
Cooking time: 0 minutes
Servings: 3

Ingredients:

- 1 green onion, chopped
- 1 celery rib, chopped
- 2 eggs, hard-boiled, peeled and chopped
- 5 ounces chicken breast, roasted and chopped
- 2 tablespoons chopped parsley
- ½ tablespoons dill relish
- Salt and black pepper to the taste
- 1/3 cup mayonnaise

Directions:

In a salad bowl, mix the chicken with the eggs, celery, onion, parsley, dill, salt, pepper and mayo and serve.
Enjoy!

Nutrition: calories 253, fat 7, fiber 5, carbs 8, protein 12

Balsamic Chicken and Salad

Preparation time: 10 minutes
Cooking time: 40 minutes
Servings: 4

Ingredients:

- 1½ pound chicken breasts, skinless and boneless
- 3 tablespoons olive oil
- Salt and black pepper to the taste
- ¼ cup balsamic vinegar
- 6 ounces sweet onion, chopped
- 1 lettuce head, chopped
- 2 garlic cloves, minced
- 4 ounces mushrooms, sliced
- 1 avocado, pitted, peeled and sliced
- 3 ounces sun-dried tomatoes, chopped
- 1 orange bell pepper, sliced
- 1 teaspoon Italian seasoning
- 1 teaspoon red pepper flakes
- 1 teaspoon onion powder

Directions:

In a bowl, mix the chicken with salt, pepper, Italian seasoning, pepper flakes, onion powder and balsamic vinegar and toss. Heat up your grill over medium-high heat then add the chicken, cook for 6-7 minutes on each side and divide between plates. Heat up another pan with the oil over medium-low heat, add mushrooms, garlic, salt, pepper and onion. Stir and cook for 20 minutes. In a bowl, mix lettuce leaves with the bell pepper, sun-dried tomatoes, avocado and the mushrooms mix and add this salad next to the chicken and serve.
Enjoy!

Nutrition: calories 235, fat 13, fiber 7, carbs 15, protein 15

Meat Recipes

Pork Chops and Lemon Sauce

Preparation time: 10 minutes
Cooking time: 20 minutes
Servings: 4

Ingredients:

- 4 pork chops
- 1 cup pork rinds
- 1 egg
- ½ cup coconut cream
- 2 tablespoons olive oil
- ½ cup chicken stock
- 3 tablespoons lemon juice
- A pinch of salt and black pepper
- 2 tablespoons chopped chives

Directions:
In a bowl, whisk the egg with salt and pepper. Put the pork rinds in another bowl. Dip pork chops in egg and then in pork rinds. Heat up a pan with the oil over medium-high heat and add the coated pork chops. Cook them for 4 minutes on one side, flip the place in the oven and cook at 400 degrees F for 10 minutes. Meanwhile, heat up a pan with the stock over medium heat, add the cream, lemon juice, salt, pepper and chives. Toss and cook for 5-6 minutes and take off the heat. Divide the pork chops between plates and drizzle the lemon sauce over the meat then serve. Enjoy!

Nutrition: calories 299, fat 7, fiber 5, carbs 13, protein 17

Pork Chops and Blackberry Sauce

Preparation time: 10 minutes
Cooking time: 15 minutes
Servings: 4

Ingredients:

- 2 pounds pork chops
- 1 teaspoon ground cinnamon
- A pinch of salt and black pepper
- 12 ounces blackberries
- ½ teaspoon dried thyme
- 2 tablespoons water
- ½ cup balsamic vinegar
- A pinch of salt and black pepper

Directions:
Season pork chops with salt and pepper and sprinkle the cinnamon and thyme all over as well. Heat up a small pot with the blackberries over medium heat. Add the vinegar, water, salt and pepper then stir, bring to a simmer and cook for 3-5 minutes. Take off the heat and brush the pork chops with half of this mix. Place the pork on the preheated grill and cook over medium heat for 6 minutes on each side. Divide the pork chops between plates, drizzle the rest of the blackberry sauce all over and serve.
Enjoy!

Nutrition: calories 261, fat 7, fiber 8, carbs 15, protein 16

Grilled Pork Chops

Preparation time: 10 minutes
Cooking time: 25 minutes
Servings: 4

Ingredients:
- 4 pork chops
- A drizzle of olive oil
- A pinch of salt and black pepper
- ½ teaspoon ground cinnamon
- ½ teaspoon sweet paprika

Directions:
In a bowl, rub the pork chops with salt, pepper, oil, cinnamon and paprika. Heat up a grill over medium-high heat, add the pork chops and cook them for 2 minutes on each side. Close the grill lid and continue to cook for 20 minutes more. Divide between plates and serve with a side salad. Enjoy!

Nutrition: calories 251, fat 6, fiber 8, carbs 14, protein 16

Rosemary Pork Chops

Preparation time: 1 hour and 10 minutes
Cooking time: 10 minutes
Servings: 4

Ingredients:
- 4 pork chops
- ¼ cup olive oil
- 2 rosemary springs
- Juice of 2 lemons
- Zest of 2 lemons
- 2 garlic cloves
- 1 teaspoon crushed red pepper
- A pinch of salt and black pepper

Directions:
In your blender, mix the oil with the rosemary, lemon juice, lemon zest, garlic and red pepper and pulse well. In a bowl, mix the pork chops with the rosemary mix, salt and pepper. Toss well and keep in the fridge for 1 hour. Place the pork chops on your preheated grill, cook for 5 minutes on each side, divide between plates and serve.
Enjoy!

Nutrition: calories 211, fat 4, fiber 4, carbs 15, protein 17

Herbed Pork Chops

Preparation time: 10 minutes
Cooking time: 10 minutes
Servings: 4

Ingredients:
- 4 pork chops, bone-in
- Zest of 1 lemon
- 3 tablespoons olive oil
- Juice of 1 lemon

- 3 garlic cloves, minced
- 1 tablespoon chopped thyme
- 1 tablespoon chopped basil
- ½ tablespoon ground black pepper

Directions:
In a bowl, mix the pork chops with lemon zest, lemon juice, oil, garlic, thyme, basil and black pepper. Mix and set aside for 10 minutes to marinate. Heat up your kitchen grill over medium-high heat, add the pork chops and cook them for 5 minutes on each side. Divide between plates and serve.
Enjoy!

Nutrition: calories 251, fat 5, fiber 9, carbs 15, protein 7

Crusted Pork Chops

Preparation time: 10 minutes
Cooking time: 14 minutes
Servings: 4

Ingredients:
- 4 pork chops, bone-in
- 2 garlic cloves, minced
- 3 tablespoons olive oil

- A pinch of salt and black pepper
- ½ cup mustard

Directions:
In a bowl, mix the garlic with the oil, salt, pepper and mustard and whisk well. Brush the pork chops with this mix and set them aside for 10 minutes. Heat up your grill over medium-high heat, add the pork chops and cook them for 6-7 minutes on each side. Divide between plates and serve.
Enjoy!

Nutrition: calories 194, fat 15, fiber 0, carbs 0, protein 15

Basil Pork Chops

Preparation time: 10 minutes
Cooking time: 12 minutes
Servings: 4

Ingredients:
- 4 pork chops
- 2 tablespoons minced garlic
- 2 tablespoons olive oil
- 1 cup minced basil
- 2 tablespoons lemon juice
- A pinch of salt and black pepper

Directions:
In a bowl, whisk the garlic with oil, basil, lemon juice, salt and pepper. Add pork chops and toss them well. Place the chops on the preheated grill over medium-high heat and cook for 6 minutes on each side. Divide between plates and serve.
Enjoy!

Nutrition: calories 261, fat 6, fiber 7, carbs 15, protein 16

Baked Pork Chops

Preparation time: 10 minutes
Cooking time: 25 minutes
Servings: 4

Ingredients:
- 4 pork chops
- 2 eggs, whisked
- ½ cup cashew meal
- 1/3 cup sunflower seeds, minced
- 2 teaspoons garlic powder
- A pinch of salt and black pepper
- 1½ teaspoon smoked paprika
- 1 teaspoon chipotle chili powder

Directions:
In a bowl, mix the cashew meal with sunflower seeds, garlic powder, salt, pepper, paprika and chili powder. Dip the pork chops in whisked eggs, then in cashew mix and place them on a lined baking sheet and bake at 400 degrees F for 25 minutes. Divide between plates and serve.
Enjoy!

Nutrition: calories 251, fat 12, fiber 4, carbs 7, protein 16

Roasted Pork Chops

Preparation time: 10 minutes
Cooking time: 15 minutes
Servings: 4

Ingredients:
- 4 pork chops, bone-in
- A pinch of salt and black pepper
- 1 tablespoon olive oil
- 6 garlic cloves, minced

Directions:
Heat up a pan with the oil over medium-high heat and add the pork chops. Season with salt and pepper and cook for 3 minutes. Flip the pork chops, add the garlic and place in the oven to roast at 400 degrees F for 4 minutes. Divide between plates and serve.
Enjoy!

Nutrition: calories 282, fat 12, fiber 1, carbs 6, protein 17

Skillet Pork Chops

Preparation time: 10 minutes
Cooking time: 25 minutes
Servings: 6

Ingredients:
- 6 pork chops, bone-in
- 3 tablespoons olive oil
- A pinch of salt and black pepper
- ¼ teaspoon ground cumin
- ¼ teaspoon dried rosemary

Directions:
Heat up a pan with the oil over medium-high heat, add pork chops, season with salt, pepper, cumin and rosemary and cook for 5 minutes on each side. Place the pan in the oven and roast at 350 degrees F for 15 minutes. Divide between plates and serve.
Enjoy!

Nutrition: calories 261, fat 6, fiber 5, carbs 11, protein 18

Cranberry Pork

Preparation time: 10 minutes
Cooking time: 8 hours
Servings: 4

Ingredients:
- 1 ½ pounds pork roast
- ½ teaspoon fresh grated ginger
- 1 tablespoon coconut flour
- A pinch of mustard powder
- A pinch of salt and black pepper
- ½ cup cranberries
- ¼ cup water
- Juice of ½ lemon
- 2 garlic cloves, minced

Directions:
In your slow cooker, mix the roast with the ginger, flour, mustard, salt, pepper, cranberries, water, lemon juice and garlic. Cover and cook on Low for 8 hours. Slice and divide everything between plates and serve.
Enjoy!

Nutrition: calories 261, fat 4, fiber 8, carbs 9, protein 17

Spicy Pork

Preparation time: 10 minutes
Cooking time: 12 hours
Servings: 6

Ingredients:
- 6 pork chops
- 3 chipotle peppers, chopped
- ¼ cup lime juice
- 1 small yellow onion, chopped
- ¼ cup tomato paste
- 4 garlic cloves, minced
- 1½ tablespoons apple cider vinegar
- 1 teaspoon dried oregano
- 2 teaspoons ground cumin
- 1 cup chicken stock
- 1 teaspoon cloves
- 3 bay leaves

Directions:
In your slow cooker, combine the pork chops with chipotle peppers, lime juice, onion, tomato paste, garlic, vinegar, oregano, cumin, stock, cloves and bay leaves. Mix together then cover and cook on Low for 12 hours. Discard bay leaves and cloves then divide the pork mix between plates and serve.
Enjoy!

Nutrition: calories 271, fat 3, fiber 5, carbs 9, protein 16

Pork Chops and Brussels Sprouts

Preparation time: 10 minutes
Cooking time: 20 minutes
Servings: 4

Ingredients:

- 1 pound pork chops, boneless
- A pinch of salt and black pepper
- 1½ tablespoons olive oil
- 2/3 cup chicken stock
- 1 teaspoon mustard
- ½ tablespoon balsamic vinegar
- ¼ cup onion, chopped
- ¼ cup applesauce, unsweetened
- 2 garlic cloves, minced
- 1¼ cup Brussels sprouts, halved
- 1 tablespoon chopped rosemary
- 1 tablespoon chopped sage

Directions:

Heat up a pan with half of the oil over medium-high heat and add pork chops. Season with salt and pepper, cook for 6 minutes on each side and transfer to a plate. Heat up the pan again with the rest of the oil over medium heat, add stock, mustard, vinegar, onion, applesauce, garlic, rosemary and sage. Whisk well, bring to a simmer and cook for 5-6 minutes. Add Brussels sprouts, toss and cook for 4-5 minutes more. Add the pork chops, toss, cook the whole mixture for a few minutes then divide everything between plates and serve.
Enjoy!

Nutrition: calories 251, fat 6, fiber 8, carbs 12, protein 17

Braised Pork Chops

Preparation time: 10 minutes
Cooking time: 1 hour
Servings: 4

Ingredients:

- 2 tablespoons olive oil
- 4 pork chops
- A pinch of salt and black pepper
- 2 garlic cloves, minced
- 1 yellow onion, chopped
- 28 ounces canned tomatoes, chopped
- ¼ cup chicken stock
- 1 cup tomato sauce
- ¼ cup balsamic vinegar
- 1 tablespoon herbs de Provence
- 2 tablespoons chopped parsley
- 1 tablespoon chopped basil

Directions:

Heat up a pan with the oil over medium heat and add the pork chops. Season with salt and pepper, cook for 3 minutes on each side and transfer to a plate. Heat up the pan again over medium heat, add the garlic and onion, stir and cook for 10 minutes. Add tomatoes, stock, tomato sauce, vinegar, herbs and parsley, stir and cook for 10 minutes. Return the pork, also add the basil, stir, cook for 5 minutes more, divide between plates and serve.
Enjoy!

Nutrition: calories 251, fat 11, fiber 6, carbs 9, protein 16

Pork Chops and Vinegar Sauce

Preparation time: 10 minutes
Cooking time: 30 minutes
Servings: 2

Ingredients:

- 2 pork chops, boneless
- ½ cup apple cider vinegar
- 2 tablespoons olive oil
- 1 yellow onion, chopped
- 1 teaspoon fresh grated ginger
- ½ teaspoon ground cinnamon
- A pinch of salt and black pepper

Directions:

Heat up a pan with the oil over medium-high heat, add the pork chops and season with salt and pepper. Cook for 3-4 minutes on each side. Add vinegar, onion, ginger and cinnamon. Mix everything together and place in the oven to bake at 400 degrees F for 20 minutes. Divide pork chops and sauce between plates and serve.
Enjoy!

Nutrition: calories 271, fat 5, fiber 8, carbs 10, protein 17

Pork Stew

Preparation time: 10 minutes
Cooking time: 1 hour and 40 minutes
Servings: 4

Ingredients:

- 3 tablespoons olive oil
- 3 pounds pork shoulder, cubed
- 2 cups almond flour
- A pinch of salt and black pepper
- 2 yellow onions, chopped
- 2 tablespoons minced garlic
- 1 teaspoon chili pepper flakes, dried
- 4 tablespoons chopped sage
- 3 cups chicken stock
- ¼ cup tomato paste
- ½ teaspoon allspice

Directions:

In a bowl, mix the flour with salt and pepper and dredge the pork in this mix. Heat up a pot with the oil over medium-high heat, add the pork, brown for a few minutes on each side and transfer to a bowl. Add the garlic, onion, sage and pepper flakes to the pan and cook for 8 minutes. Return the pork to the pan and also add stock, allspice and tomato paste. Stir and cook everything for 1 hour and 30 minutes. Divide the stew into bowls and serve.
Enjoy!

Nutrition: calories 290, fat 8, fiber 7, carbs 12, protein 18

Pork Chili

Preparation time: 10 minutes
Cooking time: 5 hours
Servings: 6

Ingredients:

- 1 green bell pepper, chopped
- 1 pound pork, cubed
- 1 yellow onion, chopped
- 4 carrots, chopped
- Salt and black pepper to the taste
- 26 ounces canned tomatoes, chopped
- 1 teaspoon onion powder
- 1 tablespoon chopped parsley
- 4 teaspoons chili powder
- 1 teaspoon garlic powder
- 1 teaspoon sweet paprika

Directions:

Heat up a pan over medium-high heat, add meat and brown for a few minutes then transfer to your slow cooker. Add bell pepper, carrots, onions, tomatoes, salt, pepper, onion powder, parsley, chili powder, paprika and garlic powder. Stir, cover, cook on High for 5 hours then divide into bowls and serve.
Enjoy!

Nutrition: calories 274, fat 6, fiber 3, carbs 11, protein 24

Cinnamon Pork Stew

Preparation time: 10 minutes
Cooking time: 1 hour and 40 minutes
Servings: 4

Ingredients:

- 2 pounds sweet potatoes, chopped
- A drizzle of olive oil
- 1 yellow onion, chopped
- 1 pound ground pork
- 1 tablespoon chili powder
- Salt and black pepper to the taste
- 1 teaspoon ground cumin
- ½ teaspoon garlic powder
- ½ teaspoon chopped oregano
- ½ teaspoon ground cinnamon
- A pinch of cayenne pepper
- 1 bunch kale, chopped
- 2 avocados, pitted, peeled and chopped
- ½ cup chopped parsley

Directions:

Heat up a pan with the oil over medium-high heat then add sweet potatoes and onion. Stir and cook for 15 minutes then transfer to a bowl. Heat up the pan again over medium-high heat, add pork, stir and brown for a few minutes. Add salt, pepper, cumin, garlic powder, oregano, cinnamon, cayenne, water, cooked sweet potatoes, and onion. Stir and cook for 1 hour. Add kale and stir then cook for 15 minutes more. Divide into bowls and serve with avocado and parsley on top.
Enjoy!

Nutrition: calories 300, fat 7, fiber 6, carbs 19, protein 15

Pork and Peach Salad

Preparation time: 10 minutes
Cooking time: 12 minutes
Servings: 2

Ingredients:
- 2 peaches, chopped
- 3 handfuls kale, chopped
- 8 ounces pork, cut into thin strips
- 1 tablespoon olive oil
- A splash of balsamic vinegar
- Salt and black pepper to the taste

Directions:
Heat up a pan with the oil over medium-high heat, add the pork and peaches, toss and cook for 12 minutes. Transfer to a bowl, add kale, vinegar, salt and pepper, toss and serve.
Enjoy!

Nutrition: calories 260, fat 5, fiber 4, carbs 12, protein 14

Balsamic Pork Roast

Preparation time: 10 minutes
Cooking time: 8 hours
Servings: 6

Ingredients:
- 4 pound pork roast
- 6 garlic cloves, minced
- 1 yellow onion, chopped
- ½ cup balsamic vinegar
- 1 cup chicken stock
- 2 tablespoons coconut aminos
- Salt and black pepper to the taste
- A pinch of red chili pepper flakes

Directions:
In your slow cooker, mix the roast with the garlic, onion, vinegar, stock, aminos, salt, pepper and chili flakes. Mix, cover and cook on Low for 8 hours. Slice the roast, divide it between plates and serve with the cooking juices.
Enjoy!

Nutrition: calories 255, fat 7, fiber 1, carbs 12, protein 17

Pork Tenderloin with Date Gravy

Preparation time: 10 minutes
Cooking time: 40 minutes
Servings: 6

Ingredients:
- 1 ½ pounds pork tenderloin
- 2 tablespoons veggie stock
- 1/3 cup dates, pitted
- ¼ teaspoon onion powder
- ¼ teaspoon smoked paprika
- 2 tablespoons mustard
- ¼ cup coconut aminos
- Salt and black pepper to the taste

Directions:
In your food processor, mix dates with the stock, coconut aminos, mustard, paprika, salt, pepper and onion powder and blend well. Put pork tenderloin in a baking dish, drizzle the date sauce all over, toss and bake in the oven at 400 degrees F for 40 minutes. Divide between plates and serve. Enjoy!

Nutrition: calories 270, fat 8, fiber 5, carbs 13, protein 24

Pork and Apples

Preparation time: 10 minutes
Cooking time: 1 hour
Servings: 4

Ingredients:
- 1½ cups chicken stock
- Salt and black pepper to the taste
- 1 teaspoon coconut aminos
- 4 pork chops
- 1 yellow onion, chopped
- 1 tablespoon chopped thyme
- 2 garlic cloves, minced
- 2 apples, cored and sliced

Directions:
Arrange the pork chops in a roasting pan, add stock, salt, pepper, aminos, onion, thyme, garlic and apples. Mix and place in the oven and bake at 400 degrees F for 1 hour. Divide everything between plates and serve.
Enjoy!

Nutrition: calories 260, fat 12, fiber 9, carbs 14, protein 18

Paprika Pork

Preparation time: 10 minutes
Cooking time: 10 hours
Servings: 4

Ingredients:

- 5 pounds pork butt, boneless
- 1½ cups apple cider vinegar
- 1 sweet onion, chopped
- Salt and black pepper to the taste
- 2 teaspoons smoked paprika
- ½ teaspoon ground ginger
- ½ teaspoon chili powder

Directions:
In your slow cooker, mix the pork with the cider vinegar, onion, salt, pepper, paprika, ginger and chili powder. Cover and cook on Low for 10 hours. Divide everything between plates and serve. Enjoy!

Nutrition: calories 280, fat 7, fiber 8, carbs 12, protein 8

Pork and Pineapple Mix

Preparation time: 10 minutes
Cooking time: 40 minutes
Servings: 4

Ingredients:

- 8 ounces canned pineapple, crushed
- 1 tablespoon olive oil
- 1 pound ground pork
- 1 teaspoon chili powder
- 1 teaspoon garlic powder
- 1 teaspoon cumin
- Salt and black pepper to the taste
- 1 mango, chopped
- Juice of 1 lime
- 2 avocados, pitted, peeled and chopped
- ¼ cup chopped cilantro

Directions:
Heat up a pan with the oil over medium heat, add the pork, stir and brown for 3 minutes. Add garlic, cumin, chili powder, salt and pepper and stir then cook for 8 minutes. Add pineapple, mango, avocados, lime juice, cilantro, salt and pepper and stir. Cook for 5-6 minutes more then divide between plates and serve.
Enjoy!

Nutrition: calories 200, fat 6, fiber 7, carbs 12, protein 16

Pork Steaks and Pesto

Preparation time: 4 hours
Cooking time: 15 minutes
Servings: 4

Ingredients:

- ¼ cup balsamic vinegar
- 1 pound pork steaks
- ¼ cup chopped basil
- 1 tablespoons minced garlic
- 2 tablespoons olive oil
- Salt and black pepper to the taste
- 1 teaspoon onion powder

For the pesto:

- ½ cup bell peppers, roasted
- ½ cup chopped basil
- ¼ cup olive oil
- ¼ cup pine nuts
- 1 garlic clove
- Salt and black pepper to the taste

Directions:

In a bowl, mix steaks with vinegar, 2 tablespoons oil, basil, garlic, onion, salt and pepper. Toss to coat and keep in the fridge for 4 hours. Heat up a grill over medium-high heat and add the steaks, cooking for 4 minutes. Flip the steaks and cook for another 4 minutes. In your food processor, mix the basil with the roasted peppers, pine nuts, ¼ cup olive oil, garlic, salt and pepper. Pulse well and serve your steaks with the pesto on top.
Enjoy!

Nutrition: calories 270, fat 6, fiber 5, carbs 13, protein 18

Pork and Eggplant Stew

Preparation time: 10 minutes
Cooking time: 20 minutes
Servings: 4

Ingredients:

- 2 green onions, chopped
- 2 tablespoons avocado oil
- 4 garlic cloves, minced
- 1 pound ground pork
- 1 eggplant, cubed

- 14 ounces canned tomatoes, chopped
- Salt and black pepper to the taste
- 1/3 cup chopped basil
- 2 tablespoons tomato paste
- ¾ cup coconut cream

Directions:

Heat up a pan with the oil over medium heat and add garlic and onions. Stir and cook for 4 minutes. Add beef, stir and cook for 4-5 minutes more. Add eggplant, tomatoes, salt, pepper and basil, stir and cook for 5 minutes. Add tomato paste and coconut cream, stir, cook for 1 minute then divide into bowls and serve.
Enjoy!

Nutrition: calories 261, fat 11, fiber 1, carbs 8, protein 18

Pork Chops and Raspberries

Preparation time: 10 minutes
Cooking time: 20 minutes
Servings: 4

Ingredients:

- 1 cup fresh raspberries
- 1 garlic clove, minced
- 4 pork chops
- Salt and black pepper to the taste
- 1 shallot, chopped
- 1 tablespoon olive oil
- 1 tablespoon chopped cilantro

Directions:

Heat up a pan with the oil over medium-high heat, add pork chops and season with salt and pepper. Cook for 7 minutes on each side and divide between plates. Return pan to medium heat, add shallot, stir and cook for 2 minutes. Add raspberries and cilantro, stir, cook for 5 minutes, drizzle over the pork chops and serve.
Enjoy!

Nutrition: calories 250, fat 12, fiber 2, carbs 17, protein 17

Minty Pork Chops

Preparation time: 30 minutes
Cooking time: 15 minutes
Servings: 6

Ingredients:

- 8 lamb chops
- 1 cup mint leaves
- ¼ cup parsley leaves
- ¼ cup white vinegar
- ½ cup olive oil
- 2 garlic cloves, minced
- Salt and black pepper to the taste
- ¼ teaspoon red pepper flakes

Directions:

In your blender, mix mint with parsley, vinegar, oil, garlic, salt, pepper and pepper flakes, blend well and rub the pork chops with this mix and set aside for 30 minutes. Place the marinated lamb chops on the preheated grill over medium-high heat and cook for 7 minutes on each side. Divide between plates and serve with the rest of the mint sauce on top.
Enjoy!

Nutrition: calories 313, fat 19, fiber 0, carbs 21, protein 11

Pork and Zucchini Mix

Preparation time: 10 minutes
Cooking time: 20 minutes
Servings: 4

Ingredients:

- 3 tomatoes, halved
- 1 red onion, halved
- 4 pork steaks
- 2 zucchinis, sliced
- Cooking spray
- 3 tablespoons lime juice
- 1 tablespoon olive oil
- 1 jalapeno, halved and seeded
- ½ cup chopped cilantro
- 1 garlic clove, minced
- A pinch of sea salt and black pepper

Directions:

Spray a roasting pan with cooking oil, add tomatoes, zucchini, jalapeno and onion, and bake in the oven at 475 degrees F for 10 minutes. In a bowl, mix the olive oil with garlic, cilantro, lime juice, salt and black pepper. Whisk well then add to the veggies, toss and divide this between plates. Heat up a pan with some cooking spray over medium-high heat, add steaks, season them with salt and pepper and cook for 5 minutes on each side. Divide next to the veggies and serve. Enjoy!

Nutrition: calories 200, fat 5, fiber 2, carbs 10, protein 22

Pork and Beans Chili

Preparation time: 10 minutes
Cooking time: 2 hours
Servings: 8

Ingredients:

- 1 tablespoon almond flour
- 1½ tablespoon chili powder
- A pinch of cayenne pepper
- 2 teaspoons ground cumin
- A pinch of sea salt and black pepper
- 2 ¼ pounds pork loin, cubed
- 3 teaspoons olive oil
- 2 garlic cloves, minced
- 1 yellow onion, chopped
- 3 cups canned kidney beans, drained and rinsed
- 2 cups canned pinto beans, drained and rinsed
- 2 cups chopped tomatoes
- 1 cup chicken stock
- A handful parsley, chopped

Directions:

In a bowl, mix chili powder with almond flour, cayenne, cumin, salt and black pepper, stir and add the pork. Toss to coat. Heat up a pot with 2 teaspoons oil over medium-high heat, add pork, brown on all sides and transfer to a bowl. Heat up the pot with the rest of the oil over medium-high heat and add garlic and onion. Stir the mix and cook for 3 minutes. Return pork to the pot, add stock, kidney beans, pinto beans and tomatoes, stir and bring to a boil. Reduce heat to medium, cover and cook for 1 hour and 45 minutes. Add the parsley, stir, divide into bowls and serve.
Enjoy!

Nutrition: calories 291, fat 4, fiber 10, carbs 15, protein 24

Thai Pork Stir Fry

Preparation time: 10 minutes
Cooking time: 10 minutes
Servings: 4

Ingredients:

- 1 tablespoon rice vinegar
- 4 ounces pork tenderloin, cut into strips
- A pinch of salt and black pepper
- 1 tablespoon arrowroot powder
- 1 teaspoon fresh grated ginger
- 2 tablespoons olive oil
- 3 garlic cloves, minced
- 2 dried chili peppers, chopped
- 2 teaspoons coconut aminos
- 1 zucchini, sliced

Directions:

In a bowl, mix pork with the arrowroot, vinegar, salt, pepper and ginger. Toss to coat and set aside for 15 minutes. Heat up a pan with half of the oil over medium-high heat, add pork, salt and pepper and stir. Cook for 3 minutes, transfer to a plate and set this aside as well. Heat up the pan with the rest of the oil over medium heat, add chili peppers, garlic and zucchini pieces. Stir and cook for 1 minute. Return pork to pan, also add the aminos, stir and cook for 6-7 minutes. Divide between plates and serve.
Enjoy!

Nutrition: calories 270, fat 3, fiber 6, carbs 8, protein 15

Mexican Pork Mix

Preparation time: 10 minutes
Cooking time: 20 minutes
Servings: 4

Ingredients:

- 1 yellow onion, chopped
- 1 ½ pounds ground pork
- 2 zucchinis, roughly chopped
- 1 red bell pepper, chopped
- 28 ounces canned tomatoes, chopped
- A pinch of salt and black pepper
- 1 tablespoon chili powder

Directions:

Heat up a pan over medium heat, add the pork, stir and brown for 5 minutes. Add garlic, salt, pepper, tomatoes, bell pepper, zucchini and chili powder, stir and cook for 10 minutes. Divide into bowls and serve.
Enjoy!

Nutrition: calories 260, fat 4, fiber 5, carbs 8, protein 17

Pork and Rice Mix

Preparation time: 10 minutes
Cooking time: 20 minutes
Servings: 6

Ingredients:

- 1 pound ground pork
- 2 cups zucchinis, chopped
- ½ cup yellow onion, chopped
- A pinch of salt and black pepper
- 15 ounces canned roasted tomatoes and garlic, chopped
- 1 cup veggie stock
- 1 ½ cups brown rice

Directions:
Heat up a pan over medium-high heat, add the pork, onion, salt, pepper and zucchini, stir and cook for 7 minutes. Add the stock, tomatoes, and rice, stir and cook for 10 minutes. Divide between plates and serve.
Enjoy!

Nutrition: calories 260, fat 5, fiber 3, carbs 7, protein 12

Caraway Pork Stew

Preparation time: 10 minutes
Cooking time: 40 minutes
Servings: 6

Ingredients:

- 2 pounds pork meat, cubed
- 2 yellow onions, chopped
- 1 tablespoon olive oil
- 1 garlic clove, minced
- 3 cups chicken stock
- 2 tablespoons sweet paprika
- 1 teaspoon caraway seeds
- A pinch of salt and black pepper
- 2 tablespoons coconut flour
- 1½ cups coconut cream
- 2 tablespoons chopped dill

Directions:
Heat up a pot with the oil over medium heat, add pork and brown it for 5 minutes. Add onions and garlic, stir and cook for 5 minutes. Add stock, caraway seeds, paprika, salt and pepper, bring to a boil, cover, and cook for 30 minutes. Add coconut flour, dill and cream then stir and cook for 2-3 minutes, divide into bowls and serve.
Enjoy!

Nutrition: calories 300, fat 8, fiber 8, carbs 19, protein 16

Pork and Snow Pea Mix

Preparation time: 10 minutes
Cooking time: 20 minutes
Servings: 4

Ingredients:

- 9 ounces snow peas
- 2 tablespoons olive oil
- 1 pound pork loin, cut into thin strips
- 2 cups mushrooms, sliced
- ½ cup chopped yellow onion
- 3 tablespoons coconut cream
- A pinch of salt and black pepper

Directions:

Put snow peas in a pot, add water to cover as well as salt. Bring to a boil over medium heat, cook for 10 minutes, drain and put in a bowl.Heat up a pan with half of the oil over medium heat, add pork, a pinch of salt and pepper and cook for 5-6 minutes then transfer to a bowl.Return pan to medium heat, add the rest of the oil, the onions and mushrooms then stir and cook for 4 minutes.Add the cream, peas and pork. Stir, cook for 3 minutes and divide into bowls and serve. Enjoy!

Nutrition: calories 275, fat 4, fiber 6, carbs 7, protein 12

Pork and Turnip Stew

Preparation time: 10 minutes
Cooking time: 1 hour and 45 minutes
Servings: 4

Ingredients:

- 1 pound pork meat, cubed
- A pinch of salt and black pepper
- ¼ teaspoon smoked paprika
- 1 tablespoon olive oil
- 1½ cups water
- 1 tablespoon coconut flour
- 1 yellow onion, chopped
- ½ cup tomato sauce
- 4 turnips, cubed

Directions:

Heat up a pot with the oil over medium-high heat, add the pork mixed with the coconut flour, salt, pepper and paprika. Stir and brown for 5 minutes. Add the water, tomato sauce and onion then stir, bring to a boil, cover and simmer for 1 hour. Add the turnips and cook the stew for 45 minutes more. Divide into bowls and serve.
Enjoy!

Nutrition: calories 300, fat 7, fiber 6, carbs 10, protein 20

Pork and Leeks

Preparation time: 10 minutes
Cooking time: 1 hour and 15 minutes
Servings: 4

Ingredients:

- 2 pounds pork, cubed
- 2 carrots, chopped
- 3 leek, chopped
- 1 celery stalk, chopped
- 1 teaspoon black peppercorns
- 2 yellow onions, chopped
- 1 tablespoon chopped parsley
- 2 cups coconut cream
- 1 teaspoon mustard
- A pinch of salt and black pepper

Directions:
Put the pork in a pot, add peppercorns, leeks, carrots, celery, onions and water to cover. Bring to a boil over medium heat and cook for 1 hour stirring often. Add cream, mustard, salt and pepper, stir, cook for 15 minutes then divide into bowls and serve with parsley on top.
Enjoy!

Nutrition: calories 250, fat 7, fiber 7, carbs 18, protein 18

Pork Roast and Fennel

Preparation time: 10 minutes
Cooking time: 1 hour and 35 minutes
Servings: 8

Ingredients:

- 5 ½ pounds pork loin roast, trimmed and bone removed
- A pinch of salt and black pepper
- 6 garlic cloves, chopped
- 2 tablespoons chopped rosemary
- ½ cup shredded fennel
- 2 teaspoons crushed red pepper
- ¼ cup olive oil

Directions:
Place pork roast in a baking pan and season with salt and pepper. Rub with the oil and also add garlic, rosemary, fennel and red pepper. Place in the oven at 400 degrees F and bake for 1 hour. Reduce heat to 325 degrees F and bake for another 35 minutes. Carve roast into chops then divide between plates, add the fennel mix on the side and serve.
Enjoy!

Nutrition: calories 281, fat 5, fiber 7, carbs 8, protein 10

Slow Cooked Roast and Veggies

Preparation time: 10 minutes
Cooking time: 10 hours
Servings: 8

Ingredients:

- 4 pound pork roast
- 3 sweet potatoes, sliced
- 3 carrots, sliced
- 2 yellow onions, sliced
- ½ cup veggie stock
- A pinch of salt and black pepper

Directions:

In your slow cooker, mix the roast with sweet potatoes, carrots, onions, stock, salt and pepper. Toss, cover, cook on Low for 10 hours. Slice and divide everything between plates.
Enjoy!

Nutrition: calories 290, fat 4, fiber 7, carbs 10, protein 17

Pork and Papaya Salad

Preparation time: 10 minutes
Cooking time: 10 minutes
Servings: 2

Ingredients:

- 2 pork steaks
- 2 tablespoons olive oil
- 3 ½ tablespoons coconut aminos
- 4 tablespoons lime juice
- 1 big lettuce, leaves torn
- 1 cup bean sprouts
- 1 handful chopped basil
- 1 cup chopped coriander
- 1 cup papaya, peeled and chopped
- 1 cup cherry tomatoes, sliced
- A pinch of salt and cayenne pepper

Directions:

In a bowl, mix the steaks with salt, cayenne, oil and aminos. Toss and keep in the fridge for 10 minutes to marinate. Heat up a grill over medium-high heat and add steaks. Grill for 5 minutes on each side, transfer to a cutting board, cut into thin strips and put in a salad bowl. In a small pot, bring the extra marinade juices to a boil then add to the salad bowl, over the steak. Add lettuce, bean sprouts, basil, coriander, papaya and tomatoes. Toss and serve.
Enjoy!

Nutrition: calories 250, fat 5, fiber 6, carbs 21, protein 17

Pork and Bean Sprouts Soup

Preparation time: 10 minutes
Cooking time: 20 minutes
Servings: 6

Ingredients:
- ½ pound pork, cubed
- ½ pounds ground pork
- 2 tablespoons olive oil
- 5 garlic cloves, minced
- 2 stalks celery, chopped
- 3 cups clean veggie stock
- 2 scallions, chopped
- Black pepper to the taste
- ½ teaspoon ground cinnamon
- 4 tablespoons coconut aminos
- 1 cup bean sprouts
- 2 tablespoons chopped parsley
- ½ tablespoon red pepper flakes

Directions:
Heat up a large pan with the oil over medium-high heat, add pork strips, brown for 2 minutes on each side and transfer to a plate. Heat up the same pan over medium heat, add garlic, stir and cook for 1-2 minutes. Add ground pork, scallions, celery, stock, black pepper, cinnamon and aminos. Return the pork strips to the pan as well then stir, bring to a boil and cook for 15 minutes. Add bean sprouts, parsley, and pepper flakes. Toss, ladle into bowls and serve. Enjoy!

Nutrition: calories 284, fat 8, fiber 4, carbs 9, protein 15

Curry Pork

Preparation time: 30 minutes
Cooking time: 15 minutes
Servings: 8

Ingredients:
- 1 pound pork steaks, cut into strips
- ½ cup red curry paste
- 1 cup coconut milk
- 2 tablespoons coconut aminos
- 1 teaspoon ground turmeric
- 1 tablespoon olive oil
- 2 tablespoons coconut cream
- 1 cup chicken stock
- 1 tablespoon lime juice

Directions:
In a bowl, mix the pork with the red curry paste, half of the coconut milk, aminos and turmeric. Toss and keep in the fridge for 30 minutes to marinate. Heat up your kitchen grill over medium heat, add the meat, cook for 4 minutes on each side and divide between plates. Heat up a small pan over medium heat and add the coconut cream, the rest of the red curry paste and the rest of the coconut milk then stir very well. Add stock and lime juice, stir, reduce heat to low and simmer for about 10 minutes. Serve your pork with the curry sauce drizzled all over. Enjoy!

Nutrition: calories 204, fat 12, fiber 1, carbs 7, protein 16

Ground Pork Soup

Preparation time: 10 minutes
Cooking time: 30 minutes
Servings: 6

Ingredients:

- 3 garlic cloves, minced
- A drizzle of olive oil
- 8 ounces pork, ground
- A small bunch cilantro, chopped
- A pinch of salt and black pepper
- 5 tablespoons tamari sauce
- 1 egg white, whisked
- 8 cups chicken stock
- 1 stalk lemongrass, chopped
- 3 tablespoons coconut aminos
- 2 spring onions, chopped

Directions:

Heat up a pot with the oil over medium-high heat, add the pork and the garlic, stir and cook for 5 minutes. Add salt, pepper, tamari sauce, lemongrass, aminos and stock. Stir, bring to a simmer and cook over medium heat for 20 minutes. Add the spring onions and the cilantro then stir, cook for 5 minutes more, divide into bowls and serve.
Enjoy!

Nutrition: calories 290, fat 4, fiber 6, carbs 8, protein 14

Greek Pork Mix

Preparation time: 10 minutes
Cooking time: 20 minutes
Servings: 4

Ingredients:

- 3 sweet potatoes, cubed
- 1 yellow onion, chopped
- 12 mini bell peppers, chopped
- 4 medium pork steaks
- ½ cup chopped sun-dried tomatoes
- 1 tablespoon sweet paprika
- 2 tablespoons balsamic vinegar
- Juice of 1 lemon
- 1 tablespoons dried oregano
- ¼ cup olive oil
- ¼ cup kalamata olives, pitted and chopped
- 1 tablespoon chopped dill
- 2 garlic cloves, minced
- A pinch of sea salt and black pepper

Directions:

Heat up a pan with half of the oil, add the steaks and season them with salt and black pepper. Brown them for 3 minutes on each side and transfer to a baking dish. Heat up the pan again over medium-high heat, add sweet potatoes, bell peppers, tomatoes, olives and onion. Cook them for 4 minutes and add them to the baking dish as well. In a bowl, mix lemon juice with the rest of the olive oil, vinegar, garlic, paprika and oregano. Whisk well and pour over the mix in the baking dish. Place the dish in the oven at 425 degrees F and bake for 15 minutes. Divide this between plates, sprinkle the dill on top and serve.
Enjoy!

Nutrition: calories 310, fat 11, fiber 6, carbs 10, protein 21

Pork Steak and Pico de Gallo

Preparation time: 10 minutes
Cooking time: 15 minutes
Servings: 4

Ingredients:
- 2 tablespoons chili powder
- 4 medium pork steaks
- 1 teaspoon ground cumin
- ½ tablespoon sweet paprika
- 1 teaspoon onion powder
- 1 teaspoon garlic powder
- A pinch of sea salt and black pepper

For the Pico de gallo:
- 1 small red onion, chopped
- 2 tomatoes, chopped
- 2 garlic cloves, minced
- 2 tablespoons lime juice
- 1 small green bell pepper, chopped
- 1 jalapeno, chopped
- ¼ cup chopped cilantro
- ¼ teaspoon ground cumin
- Black pepper to the taste

Directions:
In a bowl, mix chili powder with a pinch of salt, black pepper, onion powder, garlic powder, paprika and 1 teaspoon cumin. Stir and rub the meat with this mix. Heat up your grill over medium-high heat, add the steaks and cook them for 6 minutes on each side then divide between plates. In a bowl, mix red onion with tomatoes, garlic, lime juice, bell pepper, jalapeno, cilantro, black pepper and ¼ teaspoon cumin. Stir, spread this over the steaks and serve.
Enjoy!

Nutrition: calories 200, fat 12, fiber 4, carbs 8, protein 12

Creamy Coconut Pork Mix

Preparation time: 10 minutes
Cooking time: 25 minutes
Servings: 4

Ingredients:
- 12 mushrooms, sliced
- 1 shallot, chopped
- 1 pound pork meat, cubed
- 2 garlic cloves, minced
- 2 tablespoons olive oil
- ¼ cup Dijon mustard
- 1 ¼ cup coconut cream
- 2 tablespoons chopped parsley
- A pinch of sea salt and black pepper

Directions:
Heat up a pan with the oil over medium-high heat, add the pork, season with salt and pepper and cook for 4 minutes on each side. Add garlic and shallots, stir and cook for 3 minutes. Add mushrooms, coconut cream, mustard, parsley, salt and black pepper. Stir, cook for 6 minutes more, divide everything into bowls and serve.
Enjoy!

Nutrition: calories 280, fat 12, fiber 6, carbs 10, protein 14

Pork Kabobs

Preparation time: 10 minutes
Cooking time: 12 minutes
Servings: 4

Ingredients:

- 2 red bell peppers, chopped
- 2 pounds pork, cubed
- 1 red onion, chopped
- 1 zucchini, sliced
- Juice of 1 lime
- 2 tablespoons chili powder
- 2 tablespoon hot sauce
- ½ tablespoons cumin powder
- ¼ cup olive oil
- ¼ cup salsa
- A pinch of sea salt and black pepper

Directions:

In a bowl, whisk the salsa with lime juice, oil, hot sauce, chili powder, cumin, salt and black pepper. Arrange the meat, bell peppers, zucchini and onion onto skewers then brush them with the salsa. Place them on the preheated grill over medium-high heat and cook them for 6 minutes on each side. Divide between plates and serve.
Enjoy!

Nutrition: calories 300, fat 5, fiber 2, carbs 12, protein 14

Pork Steaks, Potatoes and Tomatoes Mix

Preparation time: 10 minutes
Cooking time: 30 minutes
Servings: 4

Ingredients:

- 2 sweet potatoes, chopped
- 4 pork steaks
- 1 red onion, chopped
- 8 cherry tomatoes, halved
- 4 thyme springs
- 4 garlic cloves, minced
- A pinch of sea salt and black pepper
- 4 tablespoons olive oil
- ½ tablespoon sweet paprika

Directions:

In a bowl, mix oil with a pinch of salt, black pepper, garlic and paprika and stir well. Spread the sweet potatoes on a lined baking sheet and place in the oven at 425 degrees F and bake for 10 minutes. Heat up a pan over medium-high heat, add steaks and season them with salt and black pepper. Cook for 5 minutes on each side then move to the baking sheet with the veggies. Add onions and tomatoes, drizzle with the oil and garlic mix, top with thyme and bake for 15 minutes more. Divide between plates and serve.
Enjoy!

Nutrition: calories 210, fat 2, fiber 2, carbs 12, protein 10

Honey Pork Mix

Preparation time: 10 minutes
Cooking time: 20 minutes
Servings: 4

Ingredients:

- 2 green onions, chopped
- 2 tablespoons olive oil
- 1 ½ pounds pork steaks, sliced
- ¼ cup raw honey
- ½ cup coconut aminos
- 1 tablespoon fresh minced ginger
- 1 tablespoon tapioca flour
- 1 tablespoon water
- 2 garlic cloves, minced
- ¼ cup pear juice

Directions:
Heat up a pan with half of the oil over medium heat then add ginger and garlic. Stir and cook for 2 minutes. Add honey, aminos and pear juice, stir and bring to a simmer then cook for 12 minutes. Add tapioca mixed with the water, stir and cook until the mix thickens. Heat up a pan with the rest of the oil over medium-high heat and add steak slices. Brown the steaks for 4 minutes on each side. Add green onions and half of the sauce then cook for 3 minutes more. Divide everything between plates, and drizzle the rest of the sauce over the mix and serve. Enjoy!

Nutrition: calories 220, fat 8, fiber 2, carbs 12, protein 8

Parsley Pork Chops

Preparation time: 10 minutes
Cooking time: 12 minutes
Servings: 4

Ingredients:

- 3 tablespoons coconut aminos
- 4 tablespoons olive oil
- 2 tablespoons fresh grated ginger
- 4 pork chops, bone-in
- 3 tablespoons chopped parsley
- 2 garlic cloves, minced
- A pinch of sea salt and black pepper

Directions:
In a bowl, whisk oil with aminos, parsley, ginger and garlic. Place the chops on a preheated grill over medium-high heat and season them with salt and black pepper. Grill the chops for 6 minutes on each side basting them with the parsley sauce. Divide the chops between plates and serve.
Enjoy!

Nutrition: calories 260, fat 8, fiber 4, carbs 17, protein 20

Pork Steaks and Mushroom Mix

Preparation time: 30 minutes
Cooking time: 25 minutes
Servings: 2

Ingredients:

- ¼ cup olive oil
- ½ teaspoon dried oregano
- 2 garlic cloves, minced
- Juice of 1 lime
- 2 medium pork steaks
- ¼ teaspoon ground cumin
- 1 Serrano chili pepper, minced
- ¼ cup chopped cilantro
-

- A pinch of sea salt and black pepper

For the veggie mix:

- 2 red bell peppers, chopped
- 3 Portobello mushrooms, sliced
- 1 yellow onion, chopped
- 1 tablespoon olive oil
- 1 tablespoon lime juice

Directions:

In a bowl, whisk ¼ cup oil with oregano, garlic, lime juice, cumin, cilantro, chili pepper, salt and black pepper. Add the steaks and toss to coat then keep in the fridge for 30 minutes to marinate. Place steaks on the preheated grill over medium-high heat and cook for 6 minutes on each side. Divide between plates. Heat up a pan with 1 tablespoon oil over medium-high heat, add bell pepper and onion, stir and cook for 3 minutes, add mushrooms and lime juice, stir and cook for 6 minutes more. Divide next to the steaks and serve.
Enjoy!

Nutrition: calories 220, fat 6, fiber 8, carbs 14, protein 20

Slow Cooked Pork

Preparation time: 10 minutes
Cooking time: 8 hours
Servings: 4

Ingredients:

- 2 cups chicken stock
- ¼ cup raw honey
- 1 cup tomato paste
- 1 cup balsamic vinegar
- 4 pounds pork roast
- 1 tablespoon mustard

- 1 tablespoon sweet paprika
- 1 teaspoon onion powder
- 2 tablespoons chili powder
- 2 garlic cloves, minced
- Black pepper to the taste

Directions:

In your slow cooker, whisk the stock with the honey, tomato paste, vinegar, mustard, paprika, onion powder, chili powder, garlic and black pepper. Add the pork roast, toss, cover and cook on Low for 8 hours. Slice the meat, divide it and the sauce between plates and serve.
Enjoy!

Nutrition: calories 300, fat 5, fiber 2, carbs 18, protein 24

Pork and Tomato Mix

Preparation time: 2 hours
Cooking time: 12 minutes
Servings: 4

Ingredients:
- 2 teaspoons chili powder
- 1 cup crushed tomatoes
- 4 pork steaks
- 2 teaspoons onion powder
- 2 tablespoons coconut aminos
- 1 jalapeno pepper, chopped
- A pinch of sea salt and black pepper
- 1 tablespoons hot pepper
- 2 tablespoons lime juice

Directions:
In a bowl, whisk the tomatoes with hot pepper, aminos, chili powder, onion powder, salt, black pepper and lime juice. Arrange the pork in a baking dish, pour the sauce over them and set them aside for 2 hours. Set aside the tomato marinade and place the meat on the preheated grill over medium-high heat. Cook them for 6 minutes on each side basting them with the reserved marinade then divide between plates, sprinkle jalapeno on top and serve.
Enjoy!

Nutrition: calories 173, fat 5, fiber 2, carbs 9, protein 14

Pork and Mustard Sauce

Preparation time: 10 minutes
Cooking time: 12 minutes
Servings: 4

Ingredients:
- 2 garlic cloves, minced
- 1 tablespoon lemon zest
- 1 tablespoon chopped oregano
- 4 pork chops
- 2/3 cup olive oil
- 1/3 cup chopped rosemary
- 2 tablespoons balsamic vinegar
- A pinch of sea salt and black pepper
- Black pepper to the taste
- 3 tablespoons Dijon mustard

Directions:
In a bowl, whisk oil with oregano, garlic and lemon zest and brush the chops with this mix, season them with salt and pepper then place them on the preheated grill over medium-high heat and cook for 6 minutes on each side. In a separate bowl, whisk the mustard with salt, pepper, rosemary and vinegar. Divide pork chops between plates, drizzle rosemary sauce all over and serve.
Enjoy!

Nutrition: calories 217, fat 11, fiber 1, carbs 6, protein 14

Basil Ground Pork Mix

Preparation time: 10 minutes
Cooking time: 16 minutes
Servings: 4

Ingredients:

- 6 garlic cloves, minced
- 2 red chilies, chopped
- 2 tablespoons olive oil
- 1 yellow onion, chopped
- 1 ½ pounds ground pork
- A pinch of sea salt and black pepper
- 3 cups basil, chopped
- ½ cup chicken stock
- 2 cups grated carrot
- 4 tablespoons lime juice
- 2 tablespoons coconut aminos
- ½ tablespoon raw honey

Directions:
Heat up a pan with half of the oil over medium heat, add onions and a pinch of salt then stir and cook for 4 minutes. Add garlic, chili peppers, pork, and black pepper. Stir the mix and brown for 10 minutes. Add stock and half of the basil, stir and cook for 2 minutes more. In a bowl, mix the carrot with 1 tablespoon lime juice, the rest of the basil and the rest of the oil. In another bowl, mix coconut aminos with the rest of the lime juice and honey. Divide the pork and carrot mix between the plates and drizzle the honey sauce all over.
Enjoy!

Nutrition: calories 200, fat 5, fiber 5, carbs 7, protein 17

Ground Pork Skillet

Preparation time: 10 minutes
Cooking time: 30 minutes
Servings: 4

Ingredients:

- 1 pound ground pork
- 1 tablespoon parsley flakes
- 2 big tomatoes, chopped
- 2 yellow squash, cubed
- 2 green bell peppers, chopped
- 1 yellow onion, chopped
- A pinch of sea salt and black pepper

Directions:
Heat up a pan over medium-high heat, add onion and the pork then stir and cook for 10 minutes. Add tomatoes, parsley flakes, salt and black pepper. Stir and cook for 10 minutes more. Add bell pepper pieces and squash, stir, cook for 10 minutes and divide between plates and serve.
Enjoy!

Nutrition: calories 190, fat 3, fiber 4, carbs 6, protein 12

Mediterranean Bowls

Preparation time: 10 minutes
Cooking time: 25 minutes
Servings: 4

Ingredients:

- 1 pound ground pork
- 1 tablespoon olive oil
- 2 garlic cloves, minced
- 1 yellow onion, chopped
- A pinch of sea salt and black pepper
- 1 tablespoon dried parsley
- 2 tablespoons dried oregano
- 3 ounces kale, chopped
- 3 ounces endives, chopped
- ¼ cup kalamata olives, pitted and sliced
- ¼ cup green olives, pitted and sliced

Directions:
Heat up a pan with the oil over medium-high heat, add garlic, onion, salt and black pepper then stir and cook for 3 minutes. Add the pork, stir and cook for 10 minutes. Add endives, kale, oregano and parsley then cook for 5 minutes more. Add green olives and kalamata olives, stir, cook for 3-4 minutes more, divide into bowls and serve.
Enjoy!

Nutrition: calories 307, fat 7, fiber 4, carbs 9, protein 10

Pork and Greens Salad

Preparation time: 10 minutes
Cooking time: 0 minutes
Servings: 4

Ingredients:

- 1 red chili, chopped
- 2 tablespoons rice vinegar
- 1/3 cup coconut aminos
- 1 tablespoon lime juice
- 1 teaspoon olive oil
- 8 ounces mixed salad greens
- 1 tablespoon pickled ginger
- 1 red bell pepper, sliced
- 4 ounces pork, cooked and cut into thin strips

Directions:
In a salad bowl, mix the pork with red chili, vinegar, aminos, lime juice, oil, salad greens, ginger and bell pepper. Toss well and serve.
Enjoy!

Nutrition: calories 225, fat 4, fiber 4, carbs 10, protein 11

Asian Pork Mix

Preparation time: 10 minutes
Cooking time: 15 minutes
Servings: 4

Ingredients:

- Salt and black pepper to the taste
- 1½ tablespoon olive oil
- 5 scallions, chopped
- 2 tablespoons fresh grated ginger
- 2 garlic cloves, minced
- 1 pound ground pork
- 3 tablespoons coconut aminos
- 1 tablespoon chili paste
- 2 tablespoons balsamic vinegar
- 2/3 cup chicken stock
- ¼ cup chopped cilantro

Directions:

Heat up a pan with the oil over medium-high heat, add scallions, stir and cook for 1-2 minutes. Add garlic, ginger and pork, stir and cook for 6 minutes. Add chili paste, vinegar, aminos, stock, salt and pepper and stir. Cook for 5 minutes more, divide into bowls, sprinkle cilantro on top and serve.
Enjoy!

Nutrition: calories 220, fat 3, fiber 4, carbs 7, protein 12

Greek Pesto Pork

Preparation time: 20 hours
Cooking time: 8 hours
Servings: 6

Ingredients:

- 3 pounds pork shoulder boneless
- ¼ cup olive oil
- 2 teaspoons dried oregano
- ¼ cup lemon juice
- 2 teaspoons mustard
- 2 teaspoons chopped basil
- 3 garlic cloves, minced
- 2 teaspoons pesto
- Salt and black pepper to the taste

Directions:

In a bowl, whisk olive oil with lemon juice, oregano, basil, mustard, garlic, pesto, salt and pepper. Rub the pork with the marinade, cover and keep in a cold place for about a day to marinate, flipping it halfway. Transfer the meat and the marinade to your slow cooker, cover, cook on low for 8 hours. Slice and divide the meat and cooking juices between plates and serve.
Enjoy!

Nutrition: calories 300, fat 4, fiber 6, carbs 7, protein 12

Fish Recipes

Pecan Crusted Salmon

Preparation time: 20 minutes
Cooking time: 20 minutes
Servings: 6

Ingredients:

- 3 tablespoons olive oil
- 3 tablespoons mustard
- 5 teaspoons raw honey
- ½ cup chopped pecans
- 6 salmon fillets, boneless
- 3 teaspoons chopped parsley
- Salt and black pepper to the taste

Directions:

In a bowl, whisk mustard with honey and oil. In another bowl, mix the pecans with parsley and stir. Season salmon fillets with salt and pepper then place them on a baking sheet, brush with mustard mixture, top with the pecans mix and place in the oven at 400 degrees F to bake for 20 minutes. Divide between plates and serve with a side salad.
Enjoy!

Nutrition: calories 200, fat 10, fiber 5, carbs 12, protein 16

Salmon and Cauliflower

Preparation time: 10 minutes
Cooking time: 25 minutes
Servings: 4

Ingredients:

- 2 tablespoons coconut aminos
- 1 cauliflower head, florets separated and chopped
- 4 pieces salmon fillets, skinless
- 1 big red onion, cut into wedges
- 1 tablespoon olive oil
- A pinch of sea salt and black pepper

Directions:

Place the salmon in a baking dish, drizzle the oil all over and season with salt and pepper. Place in preheated broiler over medium heat and cook for about 5 minutes. Add coconut aminos, cauliflower and onion then place in the oven and bake at 400 degrees F for 15 minutes more. Divide between plates and serve.
Enjoy!

Nutrition: calories 112, fat 5, fiber 3, carbs 8, protein 7

Salmon and Black Beans

Preparation time: 10 minutes
Cooking time: 30 minutes
Servings: 4

Ingredients:

- 1 cup canned black beans, drained and rinsed
- 2 tablespoons coconut aminos
- ½ cup olive oil
- 1½ cup chicken stock
- 6 ounces salmon fillets, boneless
- 2 garlic cloves, minced
- 1 tablespoon fresh grated ginger
- 2 teaspoons white wine vinegar
- ¼ cup grated radishes
- ¼ cup grated carrots
- ¼ cup chopped scallions

Directions:

Meanwhile, in a bowl, mix the aminos with half of the oil and whisk. Cut halfway into each salmon fillet, place them in a baking dish and pour the aminos mixture all over. Toss and keep in the fridge for 10 minutes to marinate. Heat up a pan with the rest of the oil over medium heat, add garlic, ginger and black beans. Stir and cook for 3 minutes. Add vinegar and stock, stir, bring to a boil, cook for 10 minutes and divide between plates. Broil fish for 4 minutes on each side over medium-high heat then place a fillet next to the black beans and top with grated scallions, radishes and carrots.
Enjoy!

Nutrition: calories 200, fat 7, fiber 2, carbs 9, protein 9

Salmon and Roasted Pepper Mix

Preparation time: 10 minutes
Cooking time: 30 minutes
Servings: 4

Ingredients:

- 3 red onions, cut into wedges
- ¾ cup green olives, pitted
- 3 red bell peppers, roughly chopped
- ½ teaspoon smoked paprika
- Salt and black pepper to the taste
- 5 tablespoons olive oil
- 4 salmon fillets, skinless and boneless
- 2 tablespoons chopped cilantro

Directions:

Spread peppers, onions and olives on a lined baking sheet. Add smoked paprika, salt, pepper and 3 tablespoons olive oil then toss to coat. Place in the oven at 375 degrees F and bake for 15 minutes. Rub salmon fillets with the rest of the olive oil, add to the baking sheet and place in the oven to bake for 12 more minutes. Divide everything between plates, sprinkle the cilantro on top and serve.
Enjoy!

Nutrition: calories 301, fat 2, fiber 3, carbs 9, protein 12

Salmon and Black Rice

Preparation time: 10 minutes
Cooking time: 25 minutes
Servings: 2

Ingredients:

- ½ cup black rice, cooked
- 2 medium salmon fillets, skinless and boneless
- Salt and pepper to the taste
- 2 teaspoons olive oil
- 1 garlic clove, minced
- 12 ounces mixed carrots, tomato, cucumber
- 1 small mango, peeled and chopped
- 1 red chili, chopped
- 1 small piece fresh grated ginger
- Juice of 1 lime
- 1 teaspoon sesame seeds

Directions:
Season salmon fillets with salt and pepper then rub them with oil and garlic. Arrange on a lined baking sheet and place in the oven at 350 degrees F and bake for 25 minutes. In a bowl, mix carrots, tomato and cucumber with mango, lime juice, rice, ginger and chili. Mix well then divide between plates, add baked salmon on the side and serve with sesame seeds sprinkled on top. Enjoy!

Nutrition: calories 220, fat 3, fiber 3, carbs 12, protein 8

Salmon and Coconut Olive Mix

Preparation time: 10 minutes
Cooking time: 12 minutes
Servings: 4

Ingredients:

- 4 medium salmon fillets, skinless and boneless
- 1 fennel bulb, chopped
- A pinch of salt and black pepper
- ¼ cup water
- 1 cup coconut cream
- ¼ cup green olives pitted and chopped
- ¼ cup fresh chopped chives
- 1 tablespoon olive oil
- 1 tablespoon lemon juice

Directions:
Arrange the fennel in a baking dish, add salmon fillets and season with salt and black pepper. Add the water and place the mix in the microwave. Cook on High for 12 minutes then divide between plates. In a bowl, whisk the cream with chives, olives, lemon juice, olive oil, salt and black pepper. Drizzle over the salmon and fennel and serve. Enjoy!

Nutrition: calories 272, fat 4, fiber 2, carbs 12, protein 7

Mediterranean Coconut Shrimp

Preparation time: 10 minutes
Cooking time: 10 minutes
Servings: 4

Ingredients:
- 1 cup coconut cream
- 1 pound shrimp, peeled and deveined
- 1 tablespoon olive oil
- 3 garlic cloves, minced
- 1 tablespoon chopped parsley
- ¼ teaspoon hot sauce
- 1 tablespoon lemon juice
- ½ cup scallions, finely sliced

Directions:
Heat up a pan with the oil over medium-high heat, add the shrimp, toss and cook for 3 minutes. Add the garlic, the hot sauce, lemon juice and scallions. Mix and cook for 2 minutes more. Add the cream and the parsley then stir, cook for 2 minutes, divide into bowls and serve.
Enjoy!

Nutrition: calories 215, fat 3, fiber 2, carbs 8, protein 6

Smoked Salmon and Tomato Mix

Preparation time: 10 minutes
Cooking time: 0 minutes
Servings: 4

Ingredients:
- 2 tablespoons chopped scallions
- 2 tablespoons chopped sweet onion
- 1½ teaspoons lime juice
- 1 tablespoon minced chives
- 1 tablespoon olive oil
- ½ pound smoked salmon, diced
- 1 cup cherry tomatoes, halved
- Salt and black pepper to the taste
- 1 tablespoon chopped cilantro

Directions:
In a bowl, mix the salmon with tomatoes, salt, pepper, chives, onion, scallions, lime juice, oil and cilantro. Toss well and serve.
Enjoy!

Nutrition: calories 168, fat 7, fiber 3, carbs 17, protein 13

Salmon Salad with Olive Dressing

Preparation time: 10 minutes
Cooking time: 0 minutes
Servings: 4

Ingredients:

For the salad dressing:

- 3 tablespoons balsamic vinegar
- 2 tablespoons olive oil
- 1/3 cup kalamata olives, pitted and minced
- 1 garlic clove crushed and finely chopped
- Salt and black pepper to the taste
- ½ teaspoons red pepper flakes, crushed
- ½ teaspoon lemon zest

For the salad:

- 1 pound green beans, blanched and halved
- ½ pound cherry tomatoes, halved
- Salt and black pepper to the taste
- ½ fennel bulb, sliced
- ½ red onion, sliced
- 2 cups baby arugula
- ¾ pound smoked salmon, cubed

Directions:

In a bowl, whisk the vinegar with garlic, olives, oil, red pepper flakes, lemon zest, salt and pepper. In a salad bowl, mix the salmon with the beans, tomatoes, salt, pepper, fennel, onion and arugula. Add the salad dressing, toss and serve.
Enjoy!
Nutrition: calories 212, fat 3, fiber 3, carbs 6, protein 7

Mediterranean Shrimp

Preparation time: 10 minutes
Cooking time: 30 minutes
Servings: 4

Ingredients:

- 1 teaspoon lemon juice
- A pinch of salt and black pepper
- ½ cup avocado mayonnaise
- ½ teaspoon sweet paprika
- A pinch of cayenne pepper
- 3 tablespoons olive oil
- 1 fennel bulb, chopped
- 1 yellow onion, chopped
- 1 teaspoon orange zest
- 2 garlic cloves, minced
- A pinch of ground cloves
- 1 cup veggie stock
- 1 cup canned tomatoes chopped
- 1 ½ pounds big shrimp, peeled and deveined
- ¼ teaspoon saffron powder

Directions:

In a bowl, whisk the garlic with the lemon juice, mayo, cayenne, salt, black pepper, 1 tablespoon oil and paprika. Heat up a pan with the rest of the oil over medium-high heat, add onion and fennel, stir and cook for 7 minutes. Add ground cloves, stock, tomatoes, garlic mix, saffron and orange zest then stir and cook 12 minutes. Add shrimp, stir gently, simmer for 4 more minutes, divide between plates and serve.
Enjoy!
Nutrition: calories 260, fat 2, fiber 5, carbs 8, protein 4

Cod and Endive

Preparation time: 10 minutes
Cooking time: 16 minutes
Servings: 4

Ingredients:

- 4 cod fillets, boneless and skinless
- A pinch of salt and black pepper
- Juice of 1 lime
- 2 endives, shredded
- ½ teaspoon sweet paprika
- 1 tablespoon chopped cilantro
- 1 tablespoon olive oil

Directions:
Heat up a pan with the oil over medium-high heat, add the fish, season with salt and pepper and cook for 3 minutes on each side then divide between plates. Heat up the pan again over medium heat, add shredded endives, salt, pepper, lime juice and paprika. Toss and cook for 10 minutes then add next to the fish and serve with cilantro sprinkled on top.
Enjoy!

Nutrition: calories 200, fat 2, fiber 4, carbs 10, protein 8

Scallops and Cauliflower Mash

Preparation time: 10 minutes
Cooking time: 15 minutes
Servings: 4

Ingredients:

- 12 sea scallops
- 3 garlic cloves, minced
- A pinch of salt and black pepper
- 4 cups chopped cauliflower florets
- 2 tablespoons olive oil
- 1 teaspoon chopped rosemary
- ¼ cup pine nuts, toasted
- 2 cups veggie stock
- 2 tablespoons chopped spring onions

Directions:
Put stock in a pot, bring to a boil over medium-high heat, add the cauliflower, bring to a boil, reduce heat to medium, simmer for 10 minutes, drain and transfer to a blender. Add salt and pepper, pulse well then divide between plates. Heat up a pan with the oil over medium-high heat, add rosemary and garlic then stir and cook for 1 minute. Add scallops, salt and pepper and cook for 3 minutes. Add them next to the cauliflower puree, sprinkle the pine nuts and spring onions on top and serve.
Enjoy!

Nutrition: calories 211, fat 10, fiber 4, carbs 8, protein 14

Citrus Salmon

Preparation time: 10 minutes
Cooking time: 20 minutes
Servings: 8

Ingredients:

- 3 pounds salmon fillets skinless
- A pinch of salt and black pepper
- 1 tablespoon olive oil
- 2 oranges, thinly sliced
- 12 sprigs chopped parsley

Directions:

Season salmon fillet with salt and pepper and arrange in a baking dish. Top with the orange slices, drizzle the oil, sprinkle the parsley and place in the oven at 375 degrees F to bake for 20 minutes. Divide everything between plates and serve.
Enjoy!

Nutrition: calories 210, fat 6, fiber 4, carbs 8, protein 14

Smoked Trout Cakes

Preparation time: 10 minutes
Cooking time: 6 minutes
Servings: 4

Ingredients:

- 8 ounces smoked trout, skinless, boneless and flaked
- Black pepper to the taste
- Juice of ½ lime
- 1 teaspoon sriracha sauce
- 1 egg white, beaten
- 1 green onion, chopped
- 2 tablespoons coconut flour
- 1 tablespoon olive oil

Directions:

In a bowl, mix the trout with black pepper, lime juice, sriracha, onion, coconut flour and egg white. Mix well and shape into medium cakes. Heat up a pan with the oil over medium-high heat, add trout cakes, cook for 3 minutes on each side then divide between plates and serve.
Enjoy!

Nutrition: calories 209, fat 15, fiber 6, carbs 8, protein 14

Spiced Salmon

Preparation time: 10 minutes
Cooking time: 10 minutes
Servings: 2

Ingredients:

- 2 salmon fillets, boneless and skin on
- Salt and black pepper to the taste
- 1 tablespoon ground cinnamon
- 1 tablespoon coconut oil

Directions:
Heat up a pan with the coconut oil over medium heat, add cinnamon, salt and pepper and whisk. Add salmon, skin side up, and cook for 5 minutes on each side. Divide between plates and serve with a side salad.
Enjoy!

Nutrition: calories 210, fat 12, fiber 4, carbs 7, protein 14

Scallop and Strawberry Salad

Preparation time: 2 hours
Cooking time: 6 minutes
Servings: 2

Ingredients:

- 4 ounces scallops
- ½ cup Pico de gallo
- ½ cup chopped strawberries
- 1 tablespoon lime juice
- Salt and black pepper to the taste

Directions:
Heat up a pan over medium heat, add scallops, cook for 3 minutes on each side and transfer to a bowl. Add strawberries, lime juice, Pico de gallo, salt and pepper. Toss and serve cold after 2 hours.
Enjoy!

Nutrition: calories 83, fat 1, fiber 1, carbs 5, protein 14

Halibut and Fruits Salad

Preparation time: 10 minutes
Cooking time: 10 minutes
Servings: 4

Ingredients:
- 4 halibut steaks, boneless
- 1 small cucumber, chopped
- 2 kiwis, peeled and chopped
- 3 cups strawberries, halved and then sliced
- 2 tablespoons olive oil
- Juice of ½ lemon
- A pinch of sea salt and black pepper
- A pinch of cayenne pepper
- ¼ teaspoon cinnamon powder
- 1/3 cup basil, chopped
- 6 cups micro greens

Directions:
In a bowl, toss the cucumber with kiwi, strawberries, half of the oil, salt, pepper, basil, micro greens and lemon juice. Season halibut steaks with salt, pepper, cinnamon and cayenne and drizzle with the rest of the oil then rub well. Heat up a pan over medium-high heat, add the fish steaks, cook for 5 minutes on each side, divide between plates and serve with the fruity salad on the side.
Enjoy!

Nutrition: calories 270, fat 6, fiber 4, carbs 13, protein 15

Poached Cod and Leeks

Preparation time: 10 minutes
Cooking time: 20 minutes
Servings: 4

Ingredients:
- 4 cod fillets, skinless and boneless
- 2 cups veggie stock
- 2 tablespoons lemon juice
- 1 tablespoon fresh grated ginger
- 4 teaspoons lemon zest
- A pinch of sea salt and black pepper
- 3 leeks, chopped
- 2 tablespoons olive oil
- 1 pound kale, chopped
- ½ teaspoon sesame oil

Directions:
In a bowl, mix lemon zest with salt and pepper then stir and rub the fish with this mix. Heat up a pan with the stock over medium heat. Add leeks, ginger and lemon juice then stir, bring to a simmer, and cook for a few minutes. Add fish fillets to this mix, cover pan, poach the fish for 10 minutes, transfer it to a dish, strain the liquid and reserve the leeks. Heat up a pan with the olive oil over medium heat and add kale then cook for 3-4 minutes. Add strained soup and cook for 5 minutes more. Add reserved leeks, stir, cook for 2 minutes more and take off heat. Divide fish into bowls and top each fillet with the leek soup. Drizzle the sesame oil all over and serve.
Enjoy!

Nutrition: calories 278, fat 3, fiber 4, carbs 14, protein 15

Creamy Coconut Halibut

Preparation time: 10 minutes
Cooking time: 10 minutes
Servings: 4

Ingredients:
- ¼ cup coconut milk
- ¼ cup chopped cilantro
- 1 tablespoon green curry paste
- ¼ cup chopped basil
- 2 teaspoons coconut aminos
- ½ teaspoon ground turmeric
- 4 halibut fillets, boneless
- 1 tablespoon avocado oil
- 1 red chili pepper, chopped

Directions:
In your blender, puree the cilantro with coconut milk, chili pepper, basil, aminos, curry paste and turmeric. Heat up a pan with the oil over medium-high heat, add halibut fillets and cook for 4 minutes on each side. Add the coconut mix over the fish and toss gently/ Cook for 2 minutes more, divide everything between plates and serve.
Enjoy!

Nutrition: calories 210, fat 3, fiber 2, carbs 12, protein 16

Easy Baked Cod

Preparation time: 10 minutes
Cooking time: 12 minutes
Servings: 2

Ingredients:
- 2 cod fillets, boneless
- 1 garlic cloves, minced
- 1 teaspoon olive oil
- Black pepper to the taste
- 3 sun-dried tomatoes, chopped
- 1 small red onion, sliced
- ½ fennel bulb, thinly sliced
- 4 black olives, pitted and sliced
- 2 rosemary springs
- ¼ teaspoon red pepper flakes

Directions:
Grease a baking dish with the oil, add the cod, garlic, black pepper, tomatoes, onion, fennel, olives, rosemary and pepper flakes. Cover the dish, bake at 400 degrees F for 14 minutes then discard the rosemary, divide the fish and veggies between plates and serve.
Enjoy!

Nutrition: calories 260, fat 4, fiber 6, carbs 10, protein 16

Salmon with Onions

Preparation time: 10 minutes
Cooking time: 30 minutes
Servings: 2

Ingredients:

- 16 ounces pearl onions
- A drizzle of olive oil
- 2 medium salmon fillets, boneless
- 1 tablespoon dried parsley
- 1 teaspoon dried rosemary
- Black pepper to the taste

Directions:
Put the salmon in a baking dish, add the oil, parsley, rosemary and black pepper. Toss a bit, bake in the oven at 375 degrees F for 30 minutes, divide between plates and serve.
Enjoy!

Nutrition: calories 260, fat 3, fiber 3, carbs 7, protein 16

Chinese Salmon

Preparation time: 10 minutes
Cooking time: 10 minutes
Servings: 2

Ingredients:

- 2 salmon steaks
- 4 tablespoons chopped green onions
- 4 tablespoons coconut aminos
- 2 garlic cloves, minced
- 2 tablespoons olive oil
- 1 teaspoon saffron powder

Directions:
In a bowl, whisk the green onions with aminos, garlic, oil and saffron. Add the salmon steaks, toss them well, place them on the preheated grill over medium heat and cook for 5 minutes on each side. Divide between plates and serve with a side salad.
Enjoy!

Nutrition: calories 251, fat 8, fiber 2, carbs 13, protein 16

Scallops and Spinach

Preparation time: 10 minutes
Cooking time: 10 minutes
Servings: 4

Ingredients:

- 12 jumbo sea scallops
- A pinch of sea salt and black pepper
- A drizzle of olive oil
- 6 garlic cloves, minced
- 1 cup chopped yellow onion
- 12 ounces baby spinach

Directions:

Heat up the pan with the oil over medium heat then add scallops, season with salt and black pepper and cook for 3 minutes on each side then divide between plates. Heat up the pan again over medium heat, add garlic and onions, stir and cook for 3 minutes. Add spinach, toss, cook for 3 minutes more and serve next to the scallops.
Enjoy!

Nutrition: calories 206, fat 6, fiber 4, carbs 7, protein 17

Crab Salad

Preparation time: 10 minutes
Cooking time: 0 minutes
Servings: 3

Ingredients:

- 2 cups avocado, peeled, pitted and cubed
- 1 cup chopped cucumber
- 2 cups canned crab, drained and flaked
- 2 teaspoons chopped parsley
- A pinch of salt and black pepper
- ½ tablespoon olive oil
- 1 tablespoon lime juice

Directions:

In a salad bowl, mix the avocado with crab, cucumber, parsley, salt, pepper, oil and lime juice. Toss well and serve.
Enjoy!

Nutrition: calories 260, fat 17, fiber 7, carbs 11, protein 18

Cod Soup

Preparation time: 2 hours
Cooking time: 20 minutes
Servings: 4

Ingredients:

- 2 pounds cod fillets, cubed
- 10 garlic cloves, minced
- 3 tablespoons olive oil
- 1 tablespoon lemon juice
- ¼ cup chopped parsley
- 1 yellow onion, chopped
- 2 tomatoes, chopped
- 1 tablespoon tomato paste
- 2½ cups veggie stock
- A pinch of sea salt and black pepper
- 10 cherry tomatoes, halved

Directions:

In a bowl, mix 6 garlic cloves with 2 tablespoons oil, parsley, lemon juice and the fish. Toss the fish to coat then cover bowl and keep in the fridge for 2 hours to marinate. Heat up a pot with the rest of the oil over medium-high heat, add onion, stir and cook for 2 minutes. Add the rest of the garlic, tomatoes, tomato paste, stock, salt, pepper and marinated fish and mix. Bring to a simmer and cook for 10 minutes. Add cherry tomatoes, stir, cook for 6 minutes more, ladle soup into bowls and serve.
Enjoy!

Nutrition: calories 160, fat 2, fiber 2, carbs 4, protein 7

Chili Coconut Salmon

Preparation time: 10 minutes
Cooking time: 15 minutes
Servings: 6

Ingredients:

- 1 ¼ cups shredded coconut, unsweetened
- 1 pound salmon, cubed
- 1/3 cup coconut flour
- A pinch of salt and black pepper
- 1 egg
- 2 tablespoons olive oil
- ¼ cup water
- 4 red chilies, chopped
- 3 garlic cloves, minced
- ¼ cup balsamic vinegar
- ½ cup raw honey

Directions:

In a bowl, mix coconut flour with a pinch of salt and stir. In another bowl, whisk the egg with black pepper and put the shredded coconut in a third bowl. Dip salmon cubes in the coconut flour then in the egg and then in the shredded coconut mix. Heat up a pan with the oil over medium-high heat, add salmon and fry for 3 minutes on each side then divide between plates. Heat up a pan with the water over medium-high heat, add chilies, cloves, vinegar and honey. Stir, bring to a gentle boil, simmer for 4 minutes then drizzle over the salmon and serve.
Enjoy!

Nutrition: calories 211, fat 5, fiber 2, carbs 11, protein 15

Simple Clams Mix

Preparation time: 10 minutes
Cooking time: 10 minutes
Servings: 2

Ingredients:

- 3 tablespoons olive oil
- 2 pound little clams, scrubbed
- ½ teaspoon dried thyme
- 1 shallot, minced
- ½ cup veggie stock
- 2 garlic cloves, minced
- 1 apple, cored and chopped
- Juice of ½ lemon

Directions:
Heat up a pan with the oil over medium-high heat, add shallot and garlic, stir and cook for 3-4 minutes. Add the stock, clams, thyme, apple and lemon juice. Stir and cook for 6 minutes more, divide into bowls and serve.
Enjoy!

Nutrition: calories 180, fat 9, fiber 2, carbs 8, protein 10

Simple Lobster Tails

Preparation time: 10 minutes
Cooking time: 8 minutes
Servings: 4

Ingredients:

- 2 tablespoons sriracha sauce
- 4 lobster tails, cut halfway through the center
- ¼ cup coconut oil
- 1 tablespoon chopped chives
- 1 tablespoon chopped cilantro
- 1 tablespoon lemon juice
- A pinch of sea salt and black pepper

Directions:
In a bowl, whisk the oil with a pinch of salt, black pepper, lime juice, chives and sriracha sauce. Drizzle lobster tails with half of this mix then place them on heated grill over medium-high heat, cook for 4 minutes on each side and divide between plates. Pour the remaining sriracha mix over the lobster tails, sprinkle the cilantro on top and serve.
Enjoy!

Nutrition: calories 308, fat 21, fiber 6, carbs 2, protein 23

Salmon and Sun-dried Tomatoes

Preparation time: 10 minutes
Cooking time: 30 minutes
Servings: 4

Ingredients:
- 10 ounces kale, chopped
- 5 sun-dried tomatoes, chopped
- ¼ teaspoon red pepper flakes
- 4 medium salmon fillets, boneless
- A pinch of sea salt and black pepper
- 1 tablespoon olive oil
- ¼ cup chopped shallots
- 4 garlic cloves, minced

Directions:
Heat up a pan with the oil over medium-high heat, add shallots, stir and cook for 3 minutes. Add garlic, tomatoes, pepper flakes, kale, salt and pepper. Stir and cook for 4 minutes then remove from the heat. Arrange salmon fillets on a lined baking sheet, season with salt and black pepper, top with the kale mix and bake in the oven at 350 degrees F for 20 minutes. Divide between plates and serve.
Enjoy!

Nutrition: calories 210, fat 2, fiber 4, carbs 13, protein 10

Shrimp and Avocado Salad

Preparation time: 10 minutes
Cooking time: 5 minutes
Servings: 2

Ingredients:
- 1 avocado, pitted, peeled and chopped
- 1 pound shrimp, peeled and deveined
- 1 tomato, chopped
- 1 mango, peeled and chopped
- 1 jalapeno, chopped
- A drizzle of olive oil
- 1 tablespoon lime juice
- ¼ cup chopped green onions
- 4 garlic cloves, minced
- A pinch of salt and black pepper

Directions:
In a bowl, mix lime juice with jalapeno, mango, tomato, avocado and green onions. Heat up a pan with the oil over medium-high heat, add garlic then stir and cook for 2 minutes. Add shrimp, season with salt and pepper, cook for 4 minutes and divide between plates. Add the avocado salad on the side and serve.
Enjoy!

Nutrition: calories 210, fat 2, fiber 3, carbs 13, protein 8

Cod Meatballs

Preparation time: 10 minutes
Cooking time: 30 minutes
Servings: 4

Ingredients:

- A drizzle of olive oil
- 2 garlic cloves, minced
- 1/3 cup chopped onion
- 1 pound cod, boneless, skinless and minced
- ¼ cup chopped chives
- 1 egg
- A pinch of black pepper
- 2 tablespoons Dijon mustard
- 1 tablespoon coconut flour

Directions:

In a bowl, mix the cod with garlic, onion, chives, eggs, black pepper, mustard and flour. Toss together well and then shape medium meatballs out of this mix. Arrange the meatballs on a baking sheet, drizzle the olive oil over them and place in the oven at 350 degrees F. Bake for 30 minutes, divide between plates and serve with a side salad.
Enjoy!

Nutrition: calories 211, fat 5, fiber 5, carbs 6, protein 15

Trout and Chive Sauce

Preparation time: 10 minutes
Cooking time: 10 minutes
Servings: 4

Ingredients:

- 4 trout fillets, boneless
- A pinch of salt and black pepper
- 3 teaspoons lemon zest
- 3 tablespoons chopped chives
- 1 tablespoon coconut cream
- 3 tablespoons olive oil
- 2 teaspoons lemon juice

Directions:

Season trout with salt and pepper then drizzle 2 tablespoons olive oil on top, rub a bit and place the fish on the preheated grill. Cook them over medium-high heat for 4 minutes on each side and divide between plates. Heat up a pan with the rest of the oil over medium heat and add chives, lemon zest, coconut cream and lemon juice. Mix well, cook for 2 minutes then drizzle over the fish and serve.
Enjoy!

Nutrition: calories 210, fat 12, fiber 6, carbs 8, protein 20

Simple Baked Tilapia

Preparation time: 10 minutes
Cooking time: 10 minutes
Servings: 4

Ingredients:
- 4 tilapia fillets, boneless
- Salt and black pepper to the taste
- 4 tablespoons mayonnaise
- ¼ teaspoon dried basil
- ¼ teaspoon garlic powder
- 2 tablespoons lemon juice
- ¼ cup coconut oil, melted
- Cooking spray

Directions:
Spray a baking sheet with cooking spray and place tilapia on the tray. Season with salt and pepper and place in preheated broiler to cook for 3 minutes on each side. In a bowl, whisk the mayo, basil, garlic, lemon juice, onion and coconut oil then spread this over the fish. Broil for 4 minutes more, divide between plates and serve with a side salad.
Enjoy!

Nutrition: calories 215, fat 10, fiber 4, carbs 12, protein 17

Cod Curry

Preparation time: 10 minutes
Cooking time: 25 minutes
Servings: 4

Ingredients:
- 4 cod fillets, boneless
- ½ teaspoon mustard seeds
- Salt and black pepper to the taste
- 2 green chilies, chopped
- 1 teaspoon fresh grated ginger
- 1 teaspoon curry powder
- ¼ teaspoon ground cumin
- 4 tablespoons olive oil
- 1 small red onion, chopped
- 1 teaspoon ground turmeric
- ¼ cup chopped parsley
- 1½ cups coconut cream
- 3 garlic cloves, minced

Directions:
Heat up a pot with half of the oil over medium heat. Add mustard seeds and cook for 2 minutes. Add ginger, onion, garlic, turmeric, curry powder, chilies and cumin, stir and cook for 10 minutes more. Add coconut milk, salt and pepper then stir. Bring to a boil, cook for 10 minutes and take off the heat. Heat up another pan with the rest of the oil over medium heat and add fish then cook for 4 minutes. Transfer the fish on top of the curry mix, toss gently then cook for 6 more minutes. Divide between plates, sprinkle the parsley on top and serve.
Enjoy!

Nutrition: calories 210, fat 14, fiber 7, carbs 6, protein 16

Crab and Shrimp Mix

Preparation time: 10 minutes
Cooking time: 10 minutes
Servings: 4

Ingredients:

- 2 tablespoons olive oil
- 1 pound shrimp, peeled and deveined
- 1 cup crab meat
- 2 tablespoons lemon juice
- 2 tablespoons minced garlic
- 1 tablespoon lemon zest
- 1 teaspoon sweet paprika
- Salt and black pepper to the taste

Directions:

Heat up a pan with the oil over medium-high heat, add shrimp and crab then stir and cook for 3 minutes. Add garlic, paprika, lemon juice, lemon zest, salt and pepper, stir, cook for 4 minutes more, divide between plates and serve.
Enjoy!

Nutrition: calories 200, fat 3, fiber 3, carbs 11, protein 6

Italian Roasted Salmon

Preparation time: 10 minutes
Cooking time: 15 minutes
Servings: 4

Ingredients:

- 2 salmon fillets, boneless
- 2 teaspoons Italian seasoning
- ¼ cup chopped cherry tomatoes
- 1 cup chopped black olives
- 1 tablespoon lemon zest
- Salt and black pepper to the taste
- 2 tablespoons chopped cilantro
- 1 tablespoon olive oil

Directions:

Rub fish with salt, pepper, Italian seasoning and the oil and place in a baking dish. Add tomatoes, olives and lemon zest then place in the oven and bake at 400 degrees F for 15 minutes. Divide between plates and serve with chopped cilantro on top.
Enjoy!

Nutrition: calories 210, fat 7, fiber 2, carbs 11, protein 17

Stuffed Salmon

Preparation time: 10 minutes
Cooking time: 20 minutes
Servings: 2

Ingredients:

- 2 salmon fillets
- 4 teaspoons olive oil
- 5 ounces shrimp, peeled, deveined and chopped
- 6 mushrooms, chopped
- 3 green onions, chopped
- 2 cups baby spinach
- ¼ cup avocado mayonnaise
- ¼ teaspoon ground nutmeg
- ¼ cup chopped walnuts, toasted
- A pinch of salt and black pepper

Directions:
Heat up a pan with half of the oil over medium-high heat, add mushrooms, onions, salt and pepper, stir and cook for 4 minutes. Add walnuts, spinach and shrimp then stir and cook for 4 minutes. Remove from the heat and mix with the nutmeg and mayo. Make an incision lengthwise in each salmon fillet then season with salt and pepper and stuff the salmon with the shrimp mix. Heat up a pan with the rest of the oil over medium-high heat, add stuffed salmon, skin side down and cook for 2 minutes. Reduce the heat, cover, cook the fish for 10 minutes. Divide between plates and serve.
Enjoy!

Nutrition: calories 250, fat 10, fiber 3, carbs 7, protein 20

Mustard Crusted Salmon

Preparation time: 10 minutes
Cooking time: 22 minutes
Servings: 2

Ingredients:

- 2 salmon fillets, boneless
- A pinch of salt and black pepper
- 4 tablespoons mustard
- 2 tablespoons coconut oil

Directions:
Season salmon with salt and pepper and brush it with the mustard on both sides. Heat up a pan with the oil over medium-high heat, place salmon flesh side down and cook for 3 minutes on each side. Transfer to a baking dish and place in the oven at 425 degrees F to bake for 15 minutes then serve with a side salad.
Enjoy!

Nutrition: calories 240, fat 7, fiber 6, carbs 8, protein 14

Dill Haddock

Preparation time: 10 minutes
Cooking time: 30 minutes
Servings: 4

Ingredients:
- 1 pound haddock fillets
- 3 teaspoons veggie stock
- 2 tablespoons lemon juice
- Salt and black pepper to the taste
- 2 tablespoons mayonnaise
- 2 teaspoons chopped dill
- A drizzle of olive oil

Directions:
Grease a baking dish with the oil, add the fish, also add stock mixed with lemon juice, salt, pepper, mayo and dill. Toss a bit and place in the oven at 350 degrees F to bake for 30 minutes. Divide between plates and serve.
Enjoy!

Nutrition: calories 214, fat 12, fiber 4, carbs 7, protein 17

Trout and Salsa

Preparation time: 10 minutes
Cooking time: 16 minutes
Servings: 2

Ingredients:
- 2 trout fillets, boneless
- ½ cup chopped yellow onion
- 4 teaspoons olive oil
- 1 teaspoon minced garlic
- 1 green bell pepper, chopped
- ½ cup canned tomato salsa
- 2 tablespoons kalamata olives, pitted and chopped
- ¼ cup chicken stock
- A pinch of salt and black pepper

Directions:
Heat up a pan with 2 teaspoons oil over medium heat, add bell pepper and onion then stir and cook for 3 minutes. Add garlic, stock, olives and salsa, stir, cook for 5 minutes and transfer to a bowl. Heat up the pan again with the rest of the oil over medium heat, add fish, season with salt and pepper and cook for 2 minutes on each side. Transfer to a baking dish, pour the salsa over the fish and place in the oven to bake at 425 degrees F for 6 minutes. Divide between plates and serve.
Enjoy!

Nutrition: calories 200, fat 5, fiber 6, carbs 12, protein 12

Salmon Soup

Preparation time: 10 minutes
Cooking time: 30 minutes
Servings: 4

Ingredients:

- 1 red sweet bell pepper, chopped
- 2 green bell peppers, chopped
- 3 cups chicken stock
- 1 tablespoon olive oil
- 4 celery stick, chopped
- 1 brown onion, chopped
- 4 wild salmon fillets, skinless, boneless and cubed
- A pinch of sea salt and black pepper

Directions:

Heat up a pot with the oil over medium-high heat, add the onion, stir and cook for 3 minutes. Add the red and green bell pepper, stir and cook for 3 minutes more. Add the celery, salmon, salt, pepper and the stock. Toss a bit then bring to a simmer, reduce heat to medium and cook for 20 minutes. Divide into bowls and serve.
Enjoy!

Nutrition: calories 265, fat 7, fiber 5, carbs 15, protein 16

Shrimp Cakes

Preparation time: 10 minutes
Cooking time: 10 minutes
Servings: 24

Ingredients:

- ½ pound tiger shrimp, peeled, deveined and chopped
- A pinch of sea salt and black pepper
- 2 tablespoons olive oil
- ½ pound ground pork
- 1 egg, whisked
- 2 tablespoons coconut flour
- 2 tablespoons chicken stock
- 1 teaspoon coconut aminos
- 1 green onion stalk, chopped
- 1 teaspoon fresh grated ginger

Directions:

In a bowl, mix the shrimp with the pork, salt, pepper, egg, stock, aminos, onion, ginger and flour. Stir well and shape medium cakes out of this mix. Heat up a pan with the oil over medium-high heat, add the cakes and cook for 5 minutes on each side. Divide between plates and serve with a side salad.
Enjoy!

Nutrition: calories 281, fat 8, fiber 7, carbs 19, protein 8

Italian Calamari

Preparation time: 10 minutes
Cooking time: 30 minutes
Servings: 6

Ingredients:

- 15 ounces canned tomatoes, chopped
- 1½ pounds calamari, cleaned, tentacles separated and cut into thin strips
- 1 garlic clove, minced
- ½ cup veggie stock
- 1 bunch chopped parsley
- A pinch red pepper flakes
- Juice of lemon
- A drizzle of olive oil
- A pinch of sea salt and black pepper

Directions:
Heat up a pan with the oil over medium-high heat, add the garlic and pepper flakes, stir and cook for 2-3 minutes. Add calamari, stir and cook for 3 minutes more. Add tomatoes, stock, lemon juice, salt and pepper, bring to a simmer then reduce heat to medium and cook for 25 minutes. Add the parsley, stir, divide into bowls and serve.
Enjoy!

Nutrition: calories 228, fat 2, fiber 4, carbs 11, protein 39

Chili Snapper

Preparation time: 10 minutes
Cooking time: 20 minutes
Servings: 2

Ingredients:

- 2 red snapper fillets, boneless and skinless
- 3 tablespoons chili paste
- A pinch of sea salt and black pepper
- 1 tablespoon coconut aminos
- 1 garlic clove, minced
- ½ teaspoon fresh grated ginger
- 2 teaspoons sesame seeds, toasted
- 2 tablespoons olive oil
- 1 green onion, chopped
- 2 tablespoons chicken stock

Directions:
Heat up a pan with the oil over medium-high heat, add the ginger, onion and the garlic, stir and cook for 2 minutes. Add chili paste, aminos, salt, pepper and the stock, stir and cook for 3 minutes more. Add the fish fillets, toss gently and cook for 5-6 minutes on each side. Divide between plates, sprinkle sesame seeds on top and serve.
Enjoy!

Nutrition: calories 261, fat 10, fiber 7, carbs 15, protein 16

Thai Cod

Preparation time: 10 minutes
Cooking time: 10 minutes
Servings: 2

Ingredients:
- 1 tablespoon coconut aminos
- 1 cup coconut milk
- 1 tablespoon Thai curry paste
- A drizzle of olive oil
- Zest of 1 lime
- Juice of ½ lime
- 1 tablespoon fresh grated ginger
- 1 teaspoon garlic, minced
- 2 cod fillets, boneless
- 1 tablespoon chopped cilantro

Directions:
In a bowl, whisk the aminos with coconut cream, curry paste, lime zest and juice, ginger and garlic. Add the cod, toss to cover and set aside for 10 minutes to marinate. Heat up a pan with a drizzle of oil over medium heat, add the cod, cook for 5 minutes on each side, divide between plates and sprinkle cilantro on top then serve.
Enjoy!

Nutrition: calories 271, fat 4, fiber 6, carbs 14, protein 7

Cod and Peas

Preparation time: 10 minutes
Cooking time: 15 minutes
Servings: 4

Ingredients:
- 10 ounces peas, blanched
- 1 tablespoon chopped parsley
- A drizzle of olive oil
- 4 cod fillets, boneless
- 1 teaspoon dried oregano
- 2 ounces veggie stock
- 2 garlic cloves, minced
- 1 teaspoon smoked paprika
- A pinch of sea salt and black pepper

Directions:
Put parsley, paprika, oregano, stock and garlic in your food processor and blend really well. Heat up a pan with the oil over medium-high heat, add the cod, season with salt and pepper and cook for 4 minutes on each side. Add the peas and the parsley, mix and cook for 5 minutes more. Divide everything between plates and serve.
Enjoy!

Nutrition: calories 271, fat 4, fiber 6, carbs 14, protein 15

Salmon and Scallions

Preparation time: 10 minutes
Cooking time: 20 minutes
Servings: 4

Ingredients:

- 4 medium salmon fillets, boneless
- 4 scallions, chopped
- 2 tablespoons olive oil
- Zest of 1 lemon
- 1 teaspoon white vinegar
- ¼ cup chopped dill
- ¼ cup chicken stock
- A pinch of sea salt and black pepper

Directions:
Heat up a pan with half of the oil over medium-high heat, add the salmon, season with salt and pepper then cook for 6 minutes on each side and divide between plates. Heat up another pan with the rest of the oil over medium-high heat. Add scallions, stir and cook for 2 minutes. Add lemon zest, vinegar, dill, stock, salt and pepper. Stir and cook for 5 minutes more, pour over the salmon and serve.
Enjoy!

Nutrition: calories 300, fat 4, fiber 8, carbs 14, protein 17

Salmon and Carrots

Preparation time: 10 minutes
Cooking time: 15 minutes
Servings: 2

Ingredients:

- 1 tablespoon ground cinnamon
- 2 tablespoon olive oil
- 2 salmon fillets, bone-in
- 2 cups baby carrots
- 1 tablespoon lime juice
- A pinch of sea salt and black pepper

Directions:
In a bowl, mix the cinnamon with half of the oil, salt and pepper then rub the salmon with this mix. Place the salmon on the preheated grill over medium-high heat, cook for 5 minutes on each side and divide between plates. Heat up a pan with the rest of the oil over medium-high heat and add the carrots, lime juice, salt and pepper. Toss and cook for 5-6 minutes then divide next to the salmon and serve.
Enjoy!

Nutrition: calories 371, fat 26, fiber 2, carbs 6, protein 22

Chinese Mackerel

Preparation time: 10 minutes
Cooking time: 30 minutes
Servings: 4

Ingredients:
- 1 garlic clove, minced
- 1 shallot, chopped
- 1 cup chicken stock
- 2 pounds mackerel, skinless, boneless and cubed
- 1 small ginger piece, chopped
- 1 yellow onion, chopped
- 2 celery stalks, chopped
- 1 teaspoon hot mustard
- 1 tablespoon rice vinegar
- A pinch of black pepper
- A drizzle of olive oil

Directions:
Heat up a pan with the oil over medium-high heat, add the mackerel, season with black pepper and cook for 4 minutes. Add the garlic, shallot, onion, ginger and celery, toss and cook for 4 minutes more, flipping the fish as well. Add stock, mustard and vinegar, toss gently and cook for 20 minutes over medium heat. Divide into bowls and serve.
Enjoy!

Nutrition: calories 261, fat 4, fiber 8, carbs 14, protein 7

Lemony Mackerel

Preparation time: 10 minutes
Cooking time: 15 minutes
Servings: 4

Ingredients:
- Juice of 1 lemon
- Zest of 1 lemon
- 4 mackerels
- 1 tablespoon minced chives
- A pinch of sea salt and black pepper
- 2 tablespoons olive oil

Directions:
Heat up a pan with the oil over medium-high heat, add the mackerel and cook for 6 minutes on each side. Add the lemon zest, lemon juice, chives, salt and pepper then cook for 2 more minutes on each side. Divide everything between plates and serve.
Enjoy!

Nutrition: calories 289, fat 20, fiber 0, carbs 1, protein 21

French Seafood Stew

Preparation time: 10 minutes
Cooking time: 55 minutes
Servings: 6

Ingredients:
- 1 fennel bulb, sliced
- 2 thyme springs, chopped
- 1 bay leaf
- ¾ cup olive oil
- 2 shallots, chopped
- 2 yellow onions, sliced
- 3 garlic cloves, minced
- 2 tomatoes, chopped
- 1 pound sea bass, skinless, boneless and cubed
- 1 pound snapper fillets, skinless, boneless and cubed
- 1 pound shrimp, peeled and deveined
- A pinch of salt and black pepper

Directions:
Heat up a pot with the oil over medium-high heat, add shallot, onions and garlic and stir then cook for 4 minutes. Add fennel, thyme, tomatoes, bay leaf, salt and pepper, stir and cook for 5 minutes more. Add the fish and the shrimp, toss and cook for 5 minutes. Add water to cover everything and a little more salt and pepper then bring to a boil over medium heat, cover the pot and cook for 40 minutes stirring often. Remove the bay leaf then divide into bowls and serve. Enjoy!

Nutrition: calories 251, fat 4, fiber 6, carbs 14, protein 7

Scallops Stew

Preparation time: 10 minutes
Cooking time: 20 minutes
Servings: 4

Ingredients:
- 2 leeks, chopped
- 2 tablespoons olive oil
- 1 teaspoon chopped jalapeno
- 2 teaspoons chopped garlic
- A pinch of salt and black pepper
- ¼ teaspoon ground cinnamon
- 1 carrot, chopped
- 1 teaspoon ground cumin
- 1½ cups chopped tomatoes
- 1 cup veggie stock
- 1 pound shrimp, peeled and deveined
- 1 pound sea scallops
- 2 tablespoons chopped cilantro

Directions:
Heat up a pot with the oil over medium heat, add garlic and leeks, stir and cook for 7 minutes. Add jalapeno, salt, pepper, cayenne, carrots, cinnamon and cumin, stir and cook for 5 more minutes. Add tomatoes, stock, shrimp and scallops, stir, cook for 6 more minutes then divide into bowls, sprinkle cilantro on top and serve. Enjoy!

Nutrition: calories 251, fat 4, fiber 4, carbs 11, protein 17

228

Tuna Stew

Preparation time: 10 minutes
Cooking time: 35 minutes
Servings: 4

Ingredients:

- 1 yellow onion, chopped
- 1 tablespoon olive oil
- 1 garlic clove, minced
- 1 teaspoon dried chili
- ¼ pint chicken stock
- 14 ounces canned tomatoes, chopped
- 3 sweet potatoes, cubed
- 1 red pepper, chopped
- 1 teaspoon sweet paprika
- 2 tuna fillets, flaked
- 1 tablespoon chopped coriander

Directions:
Heat up a pot with the oil over medium heat, add the onions, stir and cook for 4 minutes. Add chili and garlic, stir and cook for 1 minute. Add the stock, tomatoes, potatoes, paprika and red pepper. Stir, bring to a simmer and cook for 20 minutes over medium heat. Add the tuna, cook for 10 minutes more, divide into bowls, sprinkle coriander on top and serve.
Enjoy!

Nutrition: calories 215, fat 6, fiber 7, carbs 14, protein 7

Mackerel and Tomato Stew

Preparation time: 10 minutes
Cooking time: 25 minutes
Servings: 4

Ingredients:

- 20 ounces canned tomatoes, chopped
- A pinch of chili flakes
- A pinch of salt and black pepper
- A pinch of cayenne pepper
- 2 mackerels, cleaned and halved
- 3 teaspoons olive oil
- 1 handful uziza leaves, chopped
- 1 yellow onion, chopped

Directions:
Heat up a pot with the oil over medium heat, add the onion, stir and sauté for 5 minutes. Add tomatoes, salt, pepper and cayenne, stir and cook for 5 minutes more. Add chili flakes and uziza leaves, stir and cook for 5 more minutes. Add mackerel pieces, toss gently then bring to a boil and simmer for 10 minutes. Divide the stew into bowls and serve.
Enjoy!

Nutrition: calories 179, fat 2, fiber 7, carbs 14, protein 7

Mackerel Soup

Preparation time: 10 minutes
Cooking time: 40 minutes
Servings: 4

Ingredients:

- 4 mackerel fillets, skinless, boneless and cubed
- 2 lemongrass sticks, chopped
- 1 tablespoon coconut oil
- 2 red chilies, chopped
- 12 ounces coconut milk
- 4 cups vegetable stock
- Juice of 1 lime
- A handful coriander, chopped

Directions:

Heat up a pot with the oil over medium-high heat, add lemongrass and chilies, stir and cook for 3 minutes. Add coconut milk, stock, lime juice and mackerel, stir and bring to a boil. Reduce heat to low and simmer for 35 minutes. Add coriander, stir and let the soup sit for 10 minutes. Ladle it into bowls and serve.
Enjoy!

Nutrition: calories 251, fat 7, fiber 6, carbs 10, protein 8

Scallop Chowder

Preparation time: 10 minutes
Cooking time: 15 minutes
Servings: 4

Ingredients:

- 1 pound scallops
- 2 tablespoons olive oil
- ½ cup veggie stock
- 1 bunch green onions, chopped
- A pinch of salt and black pepper
- 4 ounces mushrooms, sliced
- 2 tablespoon almond flour
- 2 tablespoons chopped parsley
- 1 cup almond milk

Directions:

Heat up a pot with the oil over medium heat, add the mushrooms and the onions, stir and cook for 4 minutes. Add the almond flour and the milk, stir and cook for 4 minutes more. Add the stock, scallops, salt and pepper then stir and cook for a final 6 minutes. Divide into bowls, sprinkle parsley on top and serve.
Enjoy!

Nutrition: calories 261, fat 12, fiber 6, carbs 14, protein 14

Scallop Cream

Preparation time: 10 minutes
Cooking time: 40 minutes
Servings: 4

Ingredients:

- 12 ounces scallops
- 3 ounces coconut cream
- 2 tablespoons avocado oil
- 1 yellow onion, chopped
- 1 pound sweet potatoes, cubed
- 1-pint chicken stock
- 10 ounces coconut milk
- 2 egg yolks
- A pinch of salt and black pepper

Directions:
Heat up a pot with the oil over medium heat, add the onion, stir and sauté for 10 minutes. Add sweet potatoes, salt and pepper, stir and cook for 10 minutes. Add the stock, bring to a simmer and cook for 10 minutes then transfer to your blender. Pulse well, return to the pot and heat everything again over medium heat. Add the scallops, stir and cook for 6 minutes more. Add the egg yolks mixed with the cream, stir, cook for 2-3 minutes more. Divide everything into bowls and serve.
Enjoy!

Nutrition: calories 251, fat 4, fiber 6, carbs 13, protein 16

Kale and Salmon Salad

Preparation time: 10 minutes
Cooking time: 0 minutes
Servings: 1

Ingredients:

- 1 carrot, grated
- A handful kale, chopped
- 1 small lettuce head, chopped
- 1 cup smoked salmon, skinless, boneless and flaked
- 1 tablespoon tahini paste
- 1 tablespoon olive oil
- A pinch of sea salt and black pepper
- Juice of ½ lime
- A pinch of chili powder

Directions:
In a salad bowl, mix the carrots with kale, lettuce and salmon. In another bowl, whisk the tahini paste with oil, salt, pepper, chili powder and lime juice. Pour over the salad, toss and serve it cold.
Enjoy!

Nutrition: calories 210, fat 6, fiber 10, carbs 14, protein 12

Summer Salmon Salad

Preparation time: 10 minutes
Cooking time: 0 minutes
Servings: 4

Ingredients:
- 1 lettuce head, torn
- A handful kale, torn
- A handful green beans
- 2 cups smoked salmon, skinless, boneless and cubed
- 2 tablespoons chopped walnuts
- 8 cherry tomatoes, halved
- 1 tablespoon lemon juice
- 8 dates, chopped
- A drizzle of olive oil

Directions:
In a salad bowl, toss the lettuce with kale, green beans, smoked salmon, tomatoes, walnuts, dates, lemon juice and oil and serve.
Enjoy!

Nutrition: calories 200, fat 4, fiber 4, carbs 9, protein 6

Purple Cabbage and Salmon Salad

Preparation time: 10 minutes
Cooking time: 0 minutes
Servings: 4

Ingredients:
- 1 purple cabbage head, shredded
- 1 cup smoked salmon, boneless, skinless and flaked
- 1 red onion, sliced
- 1 green apple, cored and chopped
- ½ cup pecans, toasted
- A handful watercress
- ½ cup olive oil
- 1 garlic clove, minced
- ¼ cup balsamic vinegar
- A pinch of sea salt and black pepper

Directions:
In a salad bowl, toss the cabbage with smoked salmon, onion, apple, pecans, watercress, garlic, salt, pepper, vinegar and oil and serve cold.
Enjoy!

Nutrition: calories 190, fat 4, fiber 5, carbs 9, protein 7

Dessert Recipes

Easy Frozen Bananas

Preparation time: 1 hour
Cooking time: 0 minutes
Servings: 12

Ingredients:
- 12 ounces dark chocolate, melted
- 3 bananas, cut into thirds
- 1 tablespoon chopped pistachios
- 1 tablespoon chopped almonds, toasted

Directions:
Thread the bananas on popsicle sticks, dip each in melted chocolate, then in almonds and pistachios. Arrange them all on a lined baking sheet and keep in the freezer for 1 hour before serving.
Enjoy!

Nutrition: calories 53, fat 2, fiber 1, carbs 10, protein 1

Watermelon Sorbet

Preparation time: 4 hours
Cooking time: 0 minutes
Servings: 10

Ingredients:
- 1 watermelon, cubed
- 1 teaspoon vanilla extract

Directions:
Arrange watermelon cubes on a baking sheet, freeze for 2 hours then transfer to a blender. Add the vanilla, pulse well then pour into a casserole dish and spread. Keep in the freezer for 2 hours more, scoop into cups and serve.
Enjoy!

Nutrition: calories 100, fat 1, fiber 3, carbs 2, protein 2

Cherry Pudding

Preparation time: 4 hours
Cooking time: 0 minutes
Servings: 12

Ingredients:
- 1 ½ cups almond milk
- ¼ cup chia seeds
- 2 tablespoons cocoa powder
- 3 tablespoons raw honey
- ½ cup cherries, pitted and sliced

Directions:
In a bowl, mix the milk with chia seeds, cocoa powder, honey and cherries, toss, leave aside covered for 4 hours in the fridge, divide into smaller cups and serve.
Enjoy!

Nutrition: calories 211, fat 2, fiber 6, carbs 12, protein 5

Apple Chips

Preparation time: 10 minutes
Cooking time: 2 hours and 30 minutes
Servings: 6

Ingredients:
- 3 apples, cored and thinly sliced
- 1 teaspoon ground cinnamon

Directions:
Spread the apple slices on a lined baking sheet, sprinkle the cinnamon all over and place in the oven to bake at 200 degrees F for 2 hours and 30 minutes. Divide the chips into bowls and serve.
Enjoy!

Nutrition: calories 100, fat 1, fiber 4, carbs 19, protein 4

Dates Bars

Preparation time: 10 minutes
Cooking time: 15 minutes
Servings: 8

Ingredients:
- 1½ cups old fashioned oats
- 5 dates, pitted
- ½ cup coconut, shredded, unsweetened
- ½ cup walnuts
- ½ teaspoon baking soda
- 2 tablespoon ground flax seeds
- 1 egg
- ¼ cup coconut oil, melted

For the dates layer:
- 1 teaspoon lemon juice
- 2 tablespoons hot water
- 18 dates, pitted

Directions:
In your food processor, mix the oats with coconut, baking soda, walnuts, 5 dates, flaxseed, oil and the egg. Pulse well and spread on a lined baking sheet. Clean the food processor, add 18 remaining dates, water and lemon juice. Puree well then spread over the crust and place in the oven to bake at 325 degrees F for 15 minutes. Cool down, slice and serve.
Enjoy!

Nutrition: calories 200, fat 6, fiber 4, carbs 22, protein 8

Avocado Brownies

Preparation time: 10 minutes
Cooking time: 25 minutes
Servings: 8

Ingredients:
- ½ cup applesauce, unsweetened
- 1 cup avocado, pitted, peeled and chopped
- ½ cup maple syrup
- 1 teaspoon vanilla extract
- ½ cup coconut flour
- 3 eggs
- ½ cup cocoa powder
- 1 teaspoon baking soda

Directions:
In your food processor, puree the applesauce with the avocado, maple syrup and vanilla then transfer to a bowl. Add flour, eggs, baking soda and cocoa powder. Stir well, pour into a lined baking dish and bake in the oven at 350 degrees F for 25 minutes, cool down, cut into squares and serve.
Enjoy!

Nutrition: calories 200, fat 3, fiber 4, carbs 12, protein 11

Roasted Rhubarb

Preparation time: 10 minutes
Cooking time: 20 minutes
Servings: 6

Ingredients:

- 9 ounces rhubarb stalks, halved
- 3 tablespoons raw honey
- ½ teaspoon vanilla extract
- 2 tablespoons orange juice
- 1 teaspoon orange zest

Directions:
Spread the rhubarb on a lined baking sheet, drizzle with honey then add vanilla, orange juice and zest. Toss and bake in the oven at 350 degrees F for 20 minutes. Divide into bowls and serve. Enjoy!

Nutrition: calories 211, fat 3, fiber 4, carbs 8, protein 7

Ginger Sweets

Preparation time: 10 minutes
Cooking time: 5 minutes
Servings: 10

Ingredients:

- 2 cups water
- 1 tablespoon ground turmeric
- ¼ cup raw honey
- 2 tablespoons lemon juice
- 4 tablespoons gelatin powder
- 1 tablespoon fresh grated ginger

Directions:
Put the water in a pot, bring to a boil over medium heat, take off the heat and whisk in honey, lemon juice, ginger and turmeric. Add the gelatin, whisk well again then pour this into a square baking dish. Leave the mix aside to cool down, cut into small squares and serve. Enjoy!

Nutrition: calories 38, fat 0, fiber 0, carbs 7, protein 3

Blueberry Cream

Preparation time: 2 hours
Cooking time: 0 minutes
Servings: 4

Ingredients:
- 9 ounces coconut cream
- 1-pint blueberries
- 2 teaspoons lemon juice

Directions:
In a bowl, mix the cream with blueberries and lemon juice. Divide into small cups and keep in the fridge for 2 hours before serving.
Enjoy!

Nutrition: calories 121, fat 4, fiber 2, carbs 9, protein 5

Orange Sorbet

Preparation time: 50 minutes
Cooking time: 0 minutes
Servings: 8

Ingredients:
- 1 pound strawberries, halved and frozen
- 1 cup orange juice

Directions:
In your food processor, mix the orange juice with the strawberries, pulse well then spread into a container. Keep in the freezer for 50 minutes then scoop into cups and serve.
Enjoy!

Nutrition: calories 121, fat 1, fiber 2, carbs 9, protein 4

Lemon Cake

Preparation time: 5 hours and 10 minutes
Cooking time: 0 minutes
Servings: 10

Ingredients:
- 2 ½ cups chopped pecans
- 1 cup dates, pitted
- ¾ cup maple syrup+ 2 tablespoons
- 3 cups cauliflower rice
- 1½ cups pineapple, crushed
- Zest of 1 lemon
- Juice of 1 lemon
- 3 avocados, pitted, peeled and halved
- ½ teaspoon lemon extract
- ½ teaspoon vanilla extract
- A pinch of ground cinnamon

Directions:
In your food processor, mix the pecans with dates, 2 tablespoons maple syrup, cauliflower rice, pineapple, lemon juice and lemon zest. Pulse well, pour into a lined cake pan and spread evenly. In your blender, mix ¾ cup maple syrup with avocados, lemon extract, vanilla and cinnamon. Pulse well, spread over the crust and keep the cake in the fridge for 5 hours. Slice and serve. Enjoy!

Nutrition: calories 215, fat 3, fiber 4, carbs 12, protein 8

Turmeric Pudding

Preparation time: 10 minutes
Cooking time: 0 minutes
Servings: 4

Ingredients:
- 1 ½ cups cashew milk
- 2 tablespoon maple syrup
- ½ cup chia seeds
- 1 teaspoon ground turmeric
- ½ teaspoon cinnamon powder
- A pinch of cardamom powder
- A pinch of cloves, ground

Directions:
In a bowl, mix the cashew milk with maple syrup, chia seeds, turmeric, cinnamon, cardamom and cloves, stir well then let set for 10 minutes. Divide into small cups and serve. Enjoy!

Nutrition: calories 199, fat 2, fiber 3, carbs 7, protein 5

Pineapple Smoothie

Preparation time: 10 minutes
Cooking time: 0 minutes
Servings: 2

Ingredients:

- 1 ½ cups pineapple chunks
- 1 cup coconut water
- 1 orange, peeled
- 1 tablespoon fresh grated ginger
- 1 teaspoon chia seeds
- 1 teaspoon ground turmeric

Directions:
In your blender, mix the pineapple with the water, orange, ginger, chia and turmeric. Pulse well, transfer to a glass and serve.
Enjoy!

Nutrition: calories 180, fat 1, fiber 6, carbs 14, protein 3

Coconut Ice Cream

Preparation time: 8 hours
Cooking time: 2 minutes
Servings: 4

Ingredients:

- 28 ounces coconut milk
- 2 tablespoons fresh grated ginger
- ¼ cup maple syrup
- 2 teaspoons ground turmeric
- ½ teaspoon ground cinnamon
- 1 teaspoon ground cardamom
- 1 teaspoon vanilla extract

Directions:
Put the milk in a small pot, add ginger, maple syrup, turmeric, cinnamon, cardamom and vanilla. Stir, heat up over medium heat for 2 minutes then transfer to a casserole dish. Spread and keep in the fridge for 5 hours. Transfer the ice cream to an ice cream machine and process for 30 minutes, then freeze for another 3 hours before serving.
Enjoy!

Nutrition: calories 200, fat 3, fiber 9, carbs 12, protein 7

Tibetan Candy

Preparation time: 10 minutes
Cooking time: 20 minutes
Servings: 12

Ingredients:

- 4 ounces almond milk
- 6 tablespoons lemon juice
- ¾ cup natural chicory root powder
- ½ cup coconut butter
- ½ cup coconut milk powder
- ¾ cup almond meal
- ¼ teaspoon ground cardamom
- 1 cup almonds
- ½ cup raisins

Directions:

In your food processor, mix the almond milk with the lemon juice, chicory root, butter, milk powder, almond meal, cardamom, almonds and raisins. Pulse well then spread on a lined baking sheet and place in the oven at 325 degrees F for 20 minutes. Allow the candies to cool down then cut into small cubes and serve.
Enjoy!

Nutrition: calories 211, fat 2, fiber 4, carbs 21, protein 7

Date Cheesecake

Preparation time: 2 hours
Cooking time: 0 minutes
Servings: 4

Ingredients:

For the crust:

- ½ cup pecans
- ½ cup macadamia nuts
- ½ cup dates
- ½ cup walnuts

For the filling:

- 1 cup date paste
- 3 cups cashews, soaked for 3 hours
- ½ cup almond milk
- 2 cups strawberries
- ¾ cup coconut oil
- ¼ cup lime juice

Directions:

Put macadamia nuts, walnuts, dates and pecans in your food processor and blend well. Spread into a cake pan and press into the bottom of the pan. Put cashews, strawberries, date paste, lime juice, almond milk and coconut oil in your food processor, blend very well then spread over the crust. Keep in the freezer for 2 hours, slice and serve.
Enjoy!

Nutrition: calories 220, fat 2, fiber 3, carbs 8, protein 2

Rhubarb Compote

Preparation time: 10 minutes
Cooking time: 5 minutes
Servings: 3

Ingredients:
- Juice of 1 lemon
- Zest of ½ orange
- 1 ½ cup maple syrup
- 4 ½ cups rhubarbs cut into medium pieces.
- 1 ½ cups water

Directions:
Put the water in a pan, add lemon juice, orange zest, maple syrup and rhubarb. Bring to a simmer over medium heat, cook for 5 minutes then divide into bowls and serve.
Enjoy!

Nutrition: calories 108, fat 1, fiber 2, carbs 4, protein 7

Sweet Green Tea and Avocado Mix

Preparation time: 4 minutes
Cooking time: 0 minutes
Servings: 4

Ingredients:
- ½ cup coconut water
- 1 ½ cup chopped avocado
- 2 tablespoons green tea powder
- 2 teaspoons lime zest
- 1 tablespoon raw honey
- 1 mango thinly, sliced

Directions:
In your blender, mix water with avocado, green tea powder, honey and lime zest. Pulse and divide into small bowls. Top with mango and serve.
Enjoy!

Nutrition: calories 225, fat 9, fiber 8, carbs 21, protein 5

Maple Ice Cream

Preparation time: 2 hours
Cooking time: 3 minutes
Servings: 8

Ingredients:

- 1 tablespoon arrowroot powder
- 2 cups coconut milk
- ¼ teaspoon vanilla extract
- 1 tablespoon water
- 1/3 cup pure maple syrup
- 1/3 cup coconut nectar

Directions:
In a small pot, mix the arrowroot with coconut milk, vanilla extract, water, maple syrup and coconut nectar. Bring to a simmer over low heat then cook for 3 minutes and transfer to a container to cool down. Keep in the freezer for 2 hours, divide into cups and serve.
Enjoy!

Nutrition: calories 176, fat 4, fiber 2, carbs 7, protein 6

Fruity Ice Cream

Preparation time: 6 hours
Cooking time: 0 minutes
Servings: 6

Ingredients:

- 1 cup chopped apples
- 1 cup chopped pineapple
- 1 cup chopped melon
- 1 cup chopped papaya
- ½ teaspoon vanilla powder
- ¾ cup cashews
- 2 tablespoons cold water

Directions:
In a blender, puree the apples with pineapple, melon, papaya, vanilla, water and cashews. Transfer to a container and keep in the freezer for 6 hours, before serving.
Enjoy!

Nutrition: calories 140, fat 1, fiber 2, carbs 9, protein 5

Coconut Cashew Fudge

Preparation time: 2 hours
Cooking time: 0 minutes
Servings: 4

Ingredients:
- 1/3 cup natural cashew butter
- 1 ½ tablespoons coconut oil
- 2 tablespoons coconut butter
- 5 tablespoons lemon juice
- ½ teaspoon lemon zest,
- 1 tablespoons maple syrup

Directions:
In a bowl, mix cashew butter with coconut butter, coconut oil, lemon juice, lemon zest and maple syrup. Stir until you obtain a creamy mix then scoop into a lined muffin tray and keep in the freezer for at least 2 hours and serve.
Enjoy!

Nutrition: calories 72, fat 4, fiber 2, carbs 8, protein 6

Goji and Hemp Bars

Preparation time: 30 minutes
Cooking time: 0 minutes
Servings: 6

Ingredients:
- ¼ cup cocoa nibs
- 1 cup almonds, soaked in water and drained
- 2 tablespoons cocoa powder
- ¼ cup hemp seeds
- ¼ cup goji berries
- ¼ cup coconut, shredded, unsweetened
- 8 dates, pitted and soaked

Directions:
In your food processor, puree the cocoa nibs with almonds, cocoa powder, hemp seeds, goji, coconut and dates.Transfer to parchment paper, spread and press it the mix down. Cut into small pieces and keep in the fridge for 30 minutes before serving.
Enjoy!

Nutrition: calories 140, fat 6, fiber 3, carbs 12, protein 9

Almond and Pomegranate Fudge

Preparation time: 2 hours
Cooking time: 5 minutes
Servings: 6

Ingredients:
- ½ cup coconut milk
- 1 teaspoon vanilla extract
- 1 ½ cups chopped dark chocolate
- ½ cup chopped almonds
- ½ cup pomegranate seeds

Directions:
Heat up the milk in a pan over medium-low heat then add the chocolate, stir and cook for 5 minutes. Add vanilla extract, pomegranate seeds and half the of the nuts, stir and pour this into a lined baking pan, spread and sprinkle with the rest of the nuts. Cover and keep in the fridge for a few hours before serving.
Enjoy!

Nutrition: calories 68, fat 1, fiber 4, carbs 6, protein 1

Cashew Cake

Preparation time: 5 hours
Cooking time: 0 minutes
Servings: 6

Ingredients:
For the crust:
- ½ cup dates, pitted
- 1 tablespoon water
- ½ teaspoon vanilla extract
- ½ cup almonds

For the cake:
- 3 cups cashews, soaked for 8 hours
- 1 cup blackberries
- ¾ cup maple syrup
- 1 tablespoon coconut oil, melted

Directions:
In your food processor, mix dates with water, vanilla and almonds and pulse well. Transfer the dough to a work surface and roll it out then transfer to a lined cake pan. In your blender, mix the maple syrup with the coconut oil, cashews and berries. Blend well, spread evenly on the crust and place cake in the freezer for 5 hours, slice and serve.
Enjoy!

Nutrition: calories 130, fat 5, fiber 5, carbs 12, protein 4

Grape Cream

Preparation time: 10 minutes
Cooking time: 0 minutes
Servings: 2

Ingredients:
- 1 pounds grapes
- ½ pound coconut cream
- A handful fresh berries for serving

Directions:
In your food processor, puree the grapes with the cream and berries. Divide into small cups and serve.
Enjoy!

Nutrition: calories 120, fat 9, fiber 3, carbs 10, protein 3

Passion Fruit Cream

Preparation time: 10 minutes
Cooking time: 50 minutes
Servings: 6

Ingredients:
- 1 cup lemon curd
- 4 passion fruits, pulp and seeds
- 3 ½ ounces maple syrup
- 3 eggs
- 2 ounces coconut oil, melted
- 3 ½ ounces almond milk
- ½ cup almond flour
- ½ teaspoon baking powder

Directions:
In a bowl, mix the lemon curd with passion fruit, maple syrup, eggs, coconut oil, milk, flour and baking powder. Stir well and divide into 6 cups. Put the cups in an oven pan, fill the pan halfway with water and place in the oven at 200 degrees F. Bake for 50 minutes, cool them down and serve.
Enjoy!

Nutrition: calories 220, fat 12, fiber 3, carbs 7, protein 8

Carrot Cake

Preparation time: 3 hours
Cooking time: 0 minutes
Servings: 6

Ingredients:

- 1 cup pineapple, dried and chopped
- 2 carrots, chopped
- 1½ cups coconut flour
- 1 cup dates, pitted
- ½ cup shredded coconut, unsweetened
- ½ teaspoon ground cinnamon

Directions:
Put carrots in your food processor, pulse then add the flour, dates, pineapple, coconut and cinnamon. Pulse again and spoon this into a cake pan, spread evenly and keep in the freezer for 3 hours before serving.
Enjoy!

Nutrition: calories 160, fat 7, fiber 4, carbs 11, protein 4.

Berries Cream

Preparation time: 20 minutes
Cooking time: 15 minutes
Servings: 4

Ingredients:

- 2 teaspoons lemon juice
- 1 pound blueberries
- 1 pound strawberries

Directions:
In a small pot, mix the lemon juice with the strawberries and blueberries. Stir, bring to a simmer over medium heat, cook for 15 minutes, divide into bowls and serve cold.
Enjoy!

Nutrition: calories 132, fat 2, fiber 3, carbs 8, protein 5

Orange and Blackberry Cream

Preparation time: 10 minutes
Cooking time: 20 minutes
Servings: 6

Ingredients:
- 5 tablespoons chicory root powder
- 1-ounce orange juice
- 1 pound blackberries

Directions:
In a pot, mix the blackberries with the orange juice and chicory powder. Stir and bring to a simmer over medium heat. Cook for 20 minutes, divide into bowls and serve cold.
Enjoy!

Nutrition: calories 110, fat 2, fiber 3, carbs 6, protein 6

Cherry Cream

Preparation time: 10 minutes
Cooking time: 15 minutes
Servings: 6

Ingredients:
- 16 ounces dark cherries, pitted and chopped
- 2 tablespoons water
- 2 tablespoons lemon juice
- 2 tablespoons chicory root powder
- ¼ teaspoon almond extract

Directions:
In a pot, mix the cherries with the water, lemon juice, chicory and almond extract. Toss and bring to a simmer over medium heat then cook for 15 minutes. Divide into cups and serve cold.
Enjoy!

Nutrition: calories 146, fat 2, fiber 2, carbs 11, protein 6

Cinnamon Apple Mix

Preparation time: 10 minutes
Cooking time: 20 minutes
Servings: 6

Ingredients:

- 6 apples, cored and roughly chopped
- 4 tablespoons chicory root powder
- 2 teaspoons vanilla extract
- 3 drops lemon oil
- 1 ½ teaspoons ground cinnamon

Directions:

In a small pot, mix the apples with chicory powder, vanilla, lemon oil and cinnamon. Stir and bring to a simmer over medium heat. Cook for 20 minutes then divide into bowls and serve cold. Enjoy!

Nutrition: calories 110, fat 2, fiber 3, carbs 5, protein 5

Mango and Nigella Seeds Stew

Preparation time: 10 minutes
Cooking time: 20 minutes
Servings: 8

Ingredients:

- 1 ½ pounds mango, peeled and cubed
- 1 teaspoon nigella seeds
- ½ cup apple cider vinegar
- 1 inch ginger, grated
- 1 tablespoon ground cinnamon
- 4 cloves

Directions:

In a small pot, combine the mango with the nigella seeds, vinegar, ginger, cinnamon and cloves. Stir, bring to a boil over medium-high heat and cook for 20 minutes. Divide into bowls and serve cold.
Enjoy!

Nutrition: calories 140, fat 2, fiber 2, carbs 8, protein 9

Blueberry Curd

Preparation time: 10 minutes
Cooking time: 15 minutes
Servings: 4

Ingredients:

- 2 tablespoons lemon juice
- 2 tablespoons sunflower oil
- 1 tablespoon chicory root powder
- 12 ounces blueberries
- 2 tablespoons flax meal mixed with 4 tablespoons water

Directions:
In a small pot, mix the blueberries with lemon juice, oil, chicory powder and flax meal. Bring to a boil over medium heat and cook for 15 minutes. Divide into bowls and serve cold.
Enjoy!

Nutrition: calories 113, fat 8, fiber 4, carbs 12, protein 1

Coconut Lemon Pudding

Preparation time: 10 minutes
Cooking time: 20 minutes
Servings: 6

Ingredients:

- 3 cups coconut milk
- Juice of 2 lemons
- Lemon zest of 2 lemons
- ½ cup maple syrup
- 3 tablespoons coconut oil, melted
- 3 tablespoons flax meal mixed with 6 tablespoons water
- 4 drops lemon oil
- 2 tablespoons gelatin
- 1 cup water

Directions:
In your blender, mix coconut milk with lemon juice, lemon zest, maple syrup, coconut oil, flax meal, lemon oil and gelatin and pulse really well. Divide this into small jars and cover with lids then place them in a water bath and place in the oven. Cook at 350 degrees F for 20 minutes then cool and serve cold.
Enjoy!

Nutrition: calories 171, fat 5, fiber 2, carbs 6, protein 8

Peaches Cream

Preparation time: 10 minutes
Cooking time: 15 minutes
Servings: 4

Ingredients:

- 4 cups water
- 3 peaches, chopped
- 2 cups rolled oats
- 1 teaspoon vanilla extract
- 2 tablespoons flax meal
- ½ cup chopped almonds

Directions:

In a small pot, combine the water with the peaches, oats, vanilla, flax meal and almonds. Stir and bring to a simmer over medium heat. Cook for 15 minutes, divide into bowls and serve cold. Enjoy!

Nutrition: calories 142, fat 3, fiber 3, carbs 7, protein 4

Simple Banana Cake

Preparation time: 10 minutes
Cooking time: 45 minutes
Servings: 4

Ingredients:

- 1 ½ cups stevia
- 2 cups almond flour
- 3 bananas, peeled and mashed
- 3 eggs
- 2 teaspoon baking powder
- 1 teaspoon ground cinnamon
- 1 teaspoon ground nutmeg

Directions:

In a bowl, mix the eggs with the stevia, baking powder, cinnamon, nutmeg, banana and flour. Stir well and pour into a greased cake pan then cover with tin foil. Place the pan in the oven, bake at 350 degrees F for 45 minutes then let the cake cool, slice and serve.
Enjoy!

Nutrition: calories 300, fat 11, fiber 11, carbs 12, protein 4

Rice Pudding

Preparation time: 10 minutes
Cooking time: 35 minutes
Servings: 4

Ingredients:
- 6 cups almond milk
- Chicory root powder to the taste
- 2 cups black rice, washed and rinsed
- 1 tablespoon ground cinnamon
- ½ cup shredded coconut, unsweetened

Directions:
In a pot, mix the rice with the milk, chicory powder, cinnamon and coconut. Bring to a simmer over medium-low heat, cook for 35 minutes, divide into bowls to chill then serve cold. Enjoy!

Nutrition: calories 170, fat 4, fiber 4, carbs 13, protein 6

Pineapple Pudding

Preparation time: 10 minutes
Cooking time: 30 minutes
Servings: 8

Ingredients:
- 1 tablespoon coconut oil, melted
- 1 cup whole rice
- 14 ounces coconut milk
- 2 eggs
- ½ teaspoon vanilla extract
- 8 ounces canned pineapple, chopped

Directions:
In a small pot, mix the oil with rice, milk, eggs, vanilla and pineapple. Stir well, bring to a simmer over medium heat and cook for 30 minutes stirring often. Divide into bowls and serve cold. Enjoy!

Nutrition: calories 172, fat 4, fiber 1, carbs 18, protein 8

Peach Marmalade

Preparation time: 10 minutes
Cooking time: 20 minutes
Servings: 6

Ingredients:
- 4 ½ cups peaches, peeled and cubed
- 2 tablespoons chicory root powder
- 1 teaspoon fresh grated ginger
- 2 cups water

Directions:
In a small pot, mix the peaches with the chicory root powder, ginger and water, stir, bring to a simmer over medium heat, cook for 20 minutes, divide into cups and serve cold.
Enjoy!

Nutrition: calories 122, fat 4, fiber 2, carbs 8, protein 2

Coconut and Cinnamon Pudding

Preparation time: 10 minutes
Cooking time: 25 minutes
Servings: 6

Ingredients:
- 2 cups coconut cream
- 1 teaspoon ground cinnamon
- 3 eggs, whisked
- Zest of 1 lemon
- ½ teaspoon ground nutmeg

Directions:
In a bowl, whisk the cream with cinnamon, eggs, lemon zest and nutmeg. Divide into small ramekins then place them in the oven, bake at 360 degrees F for 25 minutes, cool and serve cold
Enjoy!

Nutrition: calories 172, fat 15, fiber 0, carbs 3, protein 8

Apricot Cake

Preparation time: 4 hours
Cooking time: 0 minutes
Servings: 4

Ingredients:

- 12 ounces apricots, chopped
- 2 tablespoons chia seeds
- 1 tablespoon cocoa nibs
- 1 ½ tablespoon coconut oil
- 2 tablespoons almond butter

For the filling:

- 4 avocados pitted and peeled
- 5 ounces coconut oil
- 5 ounces cocoa powder
- 3 ounces maple syrup
- 2 tablespoons chicory root powder
- 1 tablespoon vanilla extract

Directions:

In your food processor blend apricots with chia seeds, cocoa nibs, 1 ½ tablespoons oil and almond butter. Spread the mix in a cake pan. In your clean food processor, mix avocados with 5 ounces coconut oil, cocoa, maple syrup, chicory root, and vanilla extract. Blend well and spread mix over cake base. Keep in the fridge for 4 hours before serving.
Enjoy!

Nutrition: calories 162, fat 11, fiber 8, carbs 10, protein 7

Simple Strawberry Pancakes

Preparation time: 10 minutes
Cooking time: 10 minutes
Servings: 4

Ingredients:

- 2 cups minced strawberries
- 2 cups almond flour
- 5 tablespoons maple syrup
- 2 ½ teaspoons baking powder
- 2 eggs, whisked
- 1 ½ cups almond milk
- Cooking spray
- 2 tablespoons almond butter, soft
- ½ teaspoon vanilla extract

Method:

In a bowl, mix the strawberries with the almond flour, syrup, baking powder, eggs, almond milk, almond butter and vanilla. Stir really well until you obtain a smooth batter. Heat up a pan over medium heat, grease with some cooking spray and add ¼ cup of batter. Spread evenly and cook for 2 minutes on each side then transfer to a plate. Repeat this with the rest of the batter and serve Enjoy!

Nutrition: calories 200, fat 2, fiber 3, carbs 5, protein 10

Blueberries Lemon Curd

Preparation time: 10 minutes
Cooking time: 10 minutes
Servings: 3

Ingredients:

- 2 cups blueberries
- ¼ cup lemon juice
- 2/3 cup stevia
- 2 teaspoons lemon zest
- 4 tablespoons coconut butter, softened
- 3 egg yolks, whisked

Directions:

Heat up a small pan over medium heat, add blueberries and lemon juice, stir and bring to a simmer. Cook for 5 minutes then strain this into a heatproof bowl and mash a bit. Put some water into a pan, bring to a simmer over medium heat and add the berries, stevia, the butter and egg yolks. Stir well, cook for a few minutes, divide into small cups and serve cold.
Enjoy!

Nutrition: calories 140, fat 6, fiber 3, carbs 12, protein 8

Coconut Rhubarb Pie

Preparation time: 30 minutes
Cooking time: 55minutes
Servings: 8

Ingredients:

- 1¼ cups almond flour
- 8 tablespoons coconut butter
- 5 tablespoons ice water

For the filling:
- 3 cups chopped rhubarb
- 1 cup maple syrup
- 3 tablespoons almond flour
- ½ teaspoon ground nutmeg
- 2 eggs, whisked
- 1 tablespoon coconut butter
- 1 pinch of salt
- 2 tablespoons almond milk

Directions:

In a bowl, mix 1¼ cups flour with 8 tablespoons coconut butter. the ice water and stir until you obtain a firm dough. Transfer dough to a floured work surface, knead it then shape into a flattened disk and wrap in plastic. Keep the dough in the fridge for 30 minutes then roll a circle and arrange in a pie pan. In a bowl, mix rhubarb with maple syrup, 3 tablespoons flour, nutmeg, eggs and milk. Stir well, pour in the pie pan and place in the oven at 400 degrees F to bake for 55 minutes then cut and serve.
Enjoy!

Nutrition: calories 200, fat 5, fiber 3, carbs 8, protein 9

Black Tea Cake

Preparation time: 10 minutes
Cooking time: 35 minutes
Servings: 10

Ingredients:

- 6 tablespoons black tea powder
- 2 cups coconut milk
- ½ cup coconut butter
- Chicory root powder to the taste
- 4 eggs
- 2 teaspoons vanilla extract
- ½ cup coconut oil
- 3 ½ cups almond flour
- 1 teaspoon baking soda
- 3 teaspoons baking powder

Directions:

Put the coconut milk in a pot and warm it up over medium heat. Add tea, stir well, take off heat and cool down. In a bowl, mix the coconut butter with the chicory powder, eggs, vanilla, coconut oil, almond flour, baking soda, baking powder and tea mix. Stir well, pour into a lined cake pan and bake in the oven at 350 degrees F for 30 minutes. Slice, divide between plates and serve. Enjoy!

Nutrition: calories 170, fat 4, fiber 5, carbs 6, protein 2

Couscous Pudding

Preparation time: 15 minutes
Cooking time: 0 minutes
Servings: 4

Ingredients:

- 1 cup couscous
- 2 tablespoons coconut water
- 2 cups natural apple juice
- 3 tablespoons coconut butter
- ¼ cup chopped pistachios
- ¼ cup chopped almonds
- 1 tablespoon ground cinnamon
- ½ cup pomegranate seeds

Directions:

In a pot, mix the couscous with the water and apple juice and bring to a boil. Cover, take off heat and set aside for 15 minutes. Uncover the pot and fluff the couscous with a fork. Add coconut butter, pistachios and almonds then stir, divide into bowls, sprinkle with cinnamon and pomegranate seeds and serve cold.
Enjoy!

Nutrition: calories 176, fat 4, fiber 5, carbs 9, protein 84

Banana and Avocado Salad

Preparation time: 10 minutes
Cooking time: 0 minutes
Servings: 4

Ingredients:
- 4 bananas, peeled and chopped
- 5 avocados, pitted, peeled and chopped
- Juice of 2 lemons
- 2 tablespoons chicory root powder

Directions:
In a bowl, mix the bananas with the avocados, lemon juice and chicory powder. Mix well and serve.
Enjoy!

Nutrition: calories 170, fat 7, fiber 5, carbs 11, protein 8

Orange and Coconut Dessert

Preparation time: 10 minutes
Cooking time: 0 minutes
Servings: 1

Ingredients:
- 1 ½ teaspoon raw honey
- 1 orange, peeled, and cut into medium segments
- 6 tablespoons coconut cream
- 4 mint leaves, chopped

Directions:
In a bowl, mix the cream with the honey, orange and mint, toss and serve cold.
Enjoy!

Nutrition: calories 150, fat 2, fiber 5, carbs 10, protein 11

Green Coconut Pudding

Preparation time: 2 hours
Cooking time: 5 minutes
Servings: 6

Ingredients:

- 14 ounces coconut milk
- 2 tablespoons green tea powder
- 14 ounces coconut cream
- 3 tablespoons chicory root powder

Directions:
Put the milk in a pan, add the chicory and green tea powder and stir. Bring to a simmer and cook for 2 minutes. Set aside to cool down then, once cool, add coconut cream, stir, divide into cups and keep in the fridge for 2 hours before serving.
Enjoy!

Nutrition: calories 220, fat 3, fiber 3, carbs 7, protein 5

Peanut Blackberry Smoothie

Preparation time: 5 minutes
Cooking time: 0 minutes
Servings: 1

Ingredients:

- ¾ cup blackberries
- 1 tablespoon peanut butter
- ¾ cup almond milk
- ½ banana, peeled
- 2 dates, pitted

Directions:
In your blender, puree the blackberries with the peanut butter, almond milk, banana and dates. Transfer to a bowl and serve cold.
Enjoy!

Nutrition: calories 120, fat 3, fiber 3, carbs 6, protein 8

Matcha and Blueberries Pudding

Preparation time: 3 hours
Cooking time: 0 minutes
Servings: 2

Ingredients:

- 2 cups almond milk
- 1 cup matcha green tea powder
- 4 tablespoons chia seeds
- 1 cup blueberries
- 1 banana, sliced

Directions:

Put chia seeds, milk and matcha powder in a bowl. Stir, cover and keep in the fridge for 3 hours. Divide into bowls, top with banana slices and blueberries and serve.
Enjoy!

Nutrition: calories 324, fat 9, fiber 18, carbs 24, protein 8

Spiced Tea Pudding

Preparation time: 10 minutes
Cooking time: 10 minutes
Servings: 3

Ingredients:

- 1 can coconut milk
- ½ cup coconut flakes
- 1 cup almond milk
- 1 teaspoon nutmeg
- 1 tablespoon ground cinnamon
- ½ teaspoon cloves
- 1 teaspoon allspice
- 1 tablespoon raw honey
- 2 teaspoons ground ginger
- 1 teaspoon cardamom
- 2 tablespoons pumpkin seeds
- 1 ½ cups berries
- 1 tablespoon chia seeds
- 1 teaspoon green tea powder

Directions:

In your blender, puree tea powder with coconut milk, almond milk, cinnamon, coconut flakes, nutmeg, allspice, cloves, honey, cardamom and ginger then divide into bowls. Heat up a pan over medium heat, add berries until bubbling then transfer to your blender and pulse well. Divide the berries into the bowls with the coconut milk mix, top with chia seeds and pumpkin seeds and serve.
Enjoy!

Nutrition: calories 150, fat 6, fiber 5, carbs 14, protein 8

Sweet Porridge Dessert

Preparation time: 10 minutes
Cooking time: 30 minutes
Servings: 4

Ingredients:
For the porridge:
- 1 ½ cups coconut milk
- ½ cup steel cut oats
- ½ cup water
- 2 black tea bags
- 1 teaspoon vanilla extract
- 2 tablespoons raw honey

For the acai berry ripple:
- 2 tablespoons acai powder
- 1 cup berries
- 1 tablespoon maple syrup

For the pistachio cream:
- ¼ cup pistachios, roasted
- ½ cup coconut milk

Directions:
Put ½ cup water in a pot and heat up over medium heat. Add oats, vanilla extract, tea bags and 1 and ½ cups coconut milk. Stir well, bring to a simmer, cover and cook for 30 minutes. Discard tea bags then add honey, stir well and take off heat. In a blender, puree 1 cup berries with acai powder and maple syrup then transfer to a bowl. In the same blender, add ½ cup coconut milk and pistachios and puree. Divide oats into bowls, add acai ripple and top with pistachios cream then serve.
Enjoy!

Nutrition: calories 140, fat 4, fiber 2, carbs 6, protein 5

Lemonade Ice Pops

Preparation time: 4 hours and 10 minutes
Cooking time: 0 minutes
Servings: 4

Ingredients:
- 2 cups cold water
- 2 iced tea and lemonade tea bags
- 1 cup hot water

Directions:
Put hot water in a bowl, add tea bags, cover and set aside for 10 minutes to steep. Squeeze the tea bags to extract all the water and then discard them. Add cold water, divide into your ice pop maker, freeze for 6 hours and serve.
Enjoy!

Nutrition: calories 38, fat 0, fiber 0, carbs 0, protein 1

Green Pudding

Preparation time: 6 hours and 5 minutes
Cooking time: 0 minutes
Servings: 4

Ingredients:
- 4 tablespoons coconut milk
- 1 cup coconut cream
- 3 tablespoons hot water
- 4 ½ teaspoons green tea powder

Directions:
In a bowl, mix green tea powder with hot water, stir well and then cool down, Add milk and cream, stir and pour into a container. Keep in the freezer for 6 hours before serving frozen. Enjoy!

Nutrition: calories 210, fat 9, fiber 5, carbs 10, protein 7

Green Tea and Chocolate Ice Cream

Preparation time: 7 hours
Cooking time: 10 minutes
Servings: 8

Ingredients:
- 2 tablespoons green tea powder
- 1 ½ cup coconut milk
- 1 ½ cups coconut cream
- 2 ounces dark chocolate, chopped

Directions:
Put the milk in a pan, heat up over medium heat then add tea powder and cream. Stir, bring to a simmer for a few minutes then take off heat and cool down. Keep in the fridge for 3 hours. Transfer mix to your ice cream maker, add chocolate then process and freeze according to directions. Freeze for 4 hours more before serving.
Enjoy!

Nutrition: calories 127, fat 11, fiber 0, carbs 3, protein 2

Avocado and Papaya Bowls

Preparation time: 10 minutes
Cooking time: 0 minutes
Servings: 1

Ingredients:

- ½ cup coconut water
- 1 ½ cup avocado, chopped
- 1 big banana, peeled and chopped
- 2 tablespoons green tea powder
- 2 teaspoons lime zest
- Melted coconut butter for serving
- 1 papaya, thinly sliced for serving

Directions:
In a bowl, mix the banana, avocado, green tea powder and lime zest. Transfer to a bowl, top with papaya and coconut butter and serve.
Enjoy!

Nutrition: calories 147, fat 2, fiber 8, carbs 10, protein 10

Easy Tea Cake

Preparation time: 10 minutes
Cooking time: 30 minutes
Servings: 12

Ingredients:

- 6 tablespoons green tea powder
- 2 cups almond milk
- 4 eggs
- 2 teaspoons vanilla extract
- 3 ½ cups almond flour
- 1 teaspoon baking soda
- 3 teaspoons baking powder

Directions:
In a bowl, mix the almond milk with green tea powder, eggs, vanilla, almond flour, baking soda and baking powder. Stir until smooth then pour into a cake pan and place in the oven to bake at 350 degrees F for 30 minutes. Slice and serve cold.
Enjoy!

Nutrition: calories 170, fat 4, fiber 9, carbs 6, protein 5

Coconut Cream

Preparation time: 2 hours
Cooking time: 5 minutes
Servings: 6

Ingredients:
- 14 ounces almond milk
- 14 ounces coconut cream
- 1 teaspoon gelatin powder

Directions:
In a pan, mix the almond milk with the cream and gelatin. Stir, bring to a simmer over medium heat and cook for 5 minutes. Divide into bowls and serve after 2 hours in the fridge.
Enjoy!

Nutrition: calories 130, fat 4, fiber 3, carbs 7, protein 4

Creamy Cantaloupe Salad

Preparation time: 5 minutes
Cooking time: 0 minutes
Servings: 1

Ingredients:
- 1-ounce coconut cream
- 6 ounces cantaloupe, peeled and cubed
- A splash of lemon juice

Directions:
In a bowl, mix the cantaloupe with the cream and lemon juice. Toss and serve.
Enjoy!

Nutrition: calories 121, fat 6, fiber 2, carbs 15, protein 2

Conclusion

An anti-inflammatory diet will improve your overall health and your appearance which sounds almost too good to be true. However, in order to get the full benefits of the diet, you need to follow the diet and stay true to all of its principles.

If you made the decision to start an anti-inflammatory diet, one of the best things you can do is start following this cookbook

With and an impressive collection of some of the best anti-inflammatory recipes, this cookbook will help you along your journey to improve your wellbeing. Along with being a fantastic source of anti-inflammatory recipes, you will also just love how everything in this cookbook tastes. There is something for everyone in here!

So, don't wait any longer! Start an anti-inflammatory diet today and start cooking some of the best anti-inflammatory dishes around using this special cookbook!

It's time to start a new life today and enjoy the all the benefits this diet can bring to you!

Recipe Index

266

13047538R00153

Made in the
USA
Monee, IL